Neurodevelopmental Pare
Psychotherapy and Mindf

This innovative book explains and introduces the use of mindfulness in therapeutic work with parents and babies, covering issues such as feeding, crying, sleeping and relating, as well as other developmental challenges which affect family life, as practiced in both clinical sessions and in the home.

The book is divided into two parts. Part 1 introduces: (1) what parent-infant psychotherapy is, its origin and evolution; (2) mindfulness, which consists in paying attention in a purposeful way in the present moment and not judgementally; and (3) the development and maturation of the brain and nervous system and how they are affected by the environment in utero and after birth. Part 2 then goes on to explore a range of topics such as parental mental illnesses, immigration, dislocation, loss, guilt, substance misuse, abuse, post-natal depression, congenital malformations and the role of fathers. It describes how these factors impact the parental relationship with, and the healthy development of the infant, drawing from relevant research to demonstrate the effectiveness of parent-infant psychotherapy and mindfulness.

The practice of psychoanalytic psychotherapy aided by mindfulness is a useful intervention for distressed families with infants, while a mindful approach to oneself and one's baby can ease parental anxiety and free-loving capacities. *Neurodevelopmental Parent-Infant Psychotherapy and Mindfulness* is an essential resource for clinicians and researchers working on parent and infant relations and will also appeal to curious new or future parents.

Maria Pozzi Monzo, born in Italy, trained in London at the Tavistock Clinic, BPF/BAP, where she now lectures. She has worked in CAMHS, PIP-UK and is currently at the School of Infant Mental Health. She is also a trainer in parent-infant psychotherapy in Italy and Switzerland. Her many publications include *The Buddha and the Baby* (2015). She was winner of the Los Angeles, Frances Tustin Memorial Prize in 1999.

"Maria Pozzi Monzo's many decades of personal meditation practice are clearly providing inspiration in her work as a parent-infant and child psychotherapist. The integration of these two fields offers a unique and valuable contribution to both disciplines, which is to be celebrated."

Ajahn Brahmavara

Neurodevelopmental Parent-Infant Psychotherapy and Mindfulness

Complementary Approaches in Work with Parents and Babies

Maria Pozzi Monzo

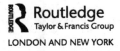
Routledge
Taylor & Francis Group

LONDON AND NEW YORK

First edition published 2020
by Routledge
2 Park Square, Milton Park, Abingdon, Oxon, OX14 4RN

and by Routledge
52 Vanderbilt Avenue, New York, NY 10017

Routledge is an imprint of the Taylor & Francis Group, an informa business

British Library Cataloguing-in-Publication Data
A catalogue record for this book is available from the British Library

Library of Congress Cataloging-in-Publication Data
Names: Monzo, Maria Pozzi, author.
Title: Neurodevelopmental parent-infant psychotherapy and
mindfulness : complementary approaches in work with parents and
babies / Maria Pozzi Monzo.
Description: First edition. | Abingdon, Oxon ; New York, NY :
Routledge, 2020. | Includes bibliographical references and index.
Identifiers: LCCN 2019035933 | ISBN 9780367429058 (hbk) | ISBN
9780367429065 (pbk) | ISBN 9781003000068 (ebk)
Subjects: LCSH: Parent-infant psychotherapy. | Mindfulness-based
cognitive therapy.
Classification: LCC RJ502.5 .M65 2020 | DDC 618.92/891425–dc23
LC record available at https://lccn.loc.gov/2019035933

ISBN: 978-0-367-42905-8 (hbk)
ISBN: 978-0-367-42906-5 (pbk)
ISBN: 978-1-003-00006-8 (ebk)

Typeset in Times New Roman
by Integra Software Services Pvt. Ltd.

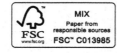

MIX
Paper from
responsible sources
FSC
www.fsc.org   FSC™ C013985

Printed in the United Kingdom
by Henry Ling Limited

I dedicate this book to my dear brother Antonio, who left us too early to be able to read it.

Contents

Foreword

I am honoured to have the opportunity to write a few words about Maria Pozzi Monzo's latest book.

As a layperson, as it were, I have first of all been able to learn easefully and accessibly about the pioneers and the current thinkers in the international field of child-infant psychotherapy.

Maria Pozzi Monzo then gives an overview of the mindfulness field which offers a full account of our current understanding and appreciation of the benefits of the many simple techniques that enable deepening awareness of the link between mind and body, leading to relaxation and well-being.

Having this wealth of information, we learn about the brain, its development in the first years of life and the effects of mindfulness practices on brain development. We learn how influential our early experiences are in setting the patterns of a lifetime and how mindfulness practices in parents can enable deep and lasting changes in early conditioning for both parents and infants. This complex area of knowledge is offered skilfully to add a further layer of appreciation for our human experience and the benefits of awareness, the mind observing the mind.

We are then privileged to be introduced to a number of case studies looking at areas of: struggle in pregnancy; early days of parenting a baby; the effects of bereavement within the family on parents and young ones; assisting the heroic struggles of parents caring for infants while afflicted with mental illness; supporting the coming to terms with and caring for a child with severe congenital disability; exploring the powerful role and influence of the father. These topics give much information and there are references to other books and resources to enable further exploration of these important areas of psychotherapeutic work with parents and infants.

The final chapter gives great hope for our shared future, as we see the resourcefulness of the human mind in its ability to let go of painful patterning and reconfigure, with professional guidance and personal effort, to more healthy and happy ways of relating. It is moving to read case studies where the lives of infants and their carers are transformed by skilful intervention and good intention at this most important time of development.

Maria Pozzi Monzo is an expert in this field and her writing is imbued with thirty-five years of hands-on experience. She conveys this in an accessible way in a book that resonates with loving kindness and compassionate interest in the many ways in which we human beings can both lose sight of our innate, peaceful presence and interconnection and can be helped with the right mix of love and methodology to re-establish these strengths and qualities in our parenting.

Maria Pozzi Monzo's many decades of personal meditation practice clearly provide inspiration in her work as a parent-infant and child psychotherapist. The integration of these two fields offers a unique and valuable contribution to both disciplines, which is to be celebrated.

Ajahn Brahmavara

Foreword

Maria Pozzi describes this book as a "writing project". She writes about her cases. And she asked the parents involved to read the pieces she wrote about them. How refreshing! This feedback gives her writing project surprising depth. Equally surprising, she attributes much of the [largely] successful outcomes of these cases to an approach called "mindfulness".

The straight forward title says it all. Dr Pozzi has given us a gem of a book about why and how mindfulness can be used in therapy sessions to better align our patients' brains and relationships and redirect development towards better outcomes. In the introduction and in each of the following ten chapters she begins with quotes from Eastern masters and ends with case presentations, with the general and the specific sandwiching a solid history and development of the relevant chapter concepts.

Her argument is straight forward. She asks us to:

- consider parent-infant psychotherapy and mindfulness offered to families in distress (Introduction) and the factors that shape the personality of the infant: epigenetics, temperament, neuropsychology, attachment style, defensive style, and sociocultural factors.
- consider parent-infant psychotherapy (Chapter 1) and Brafman's three "axioms", Winnicott's "knot", Trad's "previewing", and the impact of Bowlby's "attachment", Berg's "inner guide" and Norman (et al.)'s innovative way of creating strong emotional "links" as a bridge of transference between non-verbal infants and the analyst.
- consider mindfulness (Chapter 2) and "mindfulness-based cognitive therapy" as a way to reach, connect and balance the internal and real world workings of both head and heart, with Mindfulness-Based Cognitive Therapy (MBCT) applied to anxiety and fear, OCD, major depression and suicidality, borderline personality disorder, ADHD, PTSD, people suffering with psychosis and those managing chronic pain.
- consider the infant's brain and nervous system (Chapter 3) – with the usual host of brain parts (neurons, prefrontal cortex, amygdala, etc.) and lesser known parts as well (insula, mirror neurons) – and how the brain picks up

bodily emotions and translates them into thoughts and how mindfulness can bring changes to its functioning.

- consider pregnancy (Chapter 4) and how mothers can experience Raphael-Leff's "rebirth" and how their emotional state can produce cortisol, when under stress, which passes through the placenta and affects the birth weight of the baby.
- consider parents' guilt (Chapter 5) – unbearable, persecutory or reparative – in working with severely damaged babies.
- consider immigration (Chapter 6) dislocation and loss, Freud's distinction between melancholia and mourning, Bournes and Lewis's "replacement children", and mindfulness as a way to contain restless distress and focus the mind on breathing and bodily sensations rather than on thoughts.
- consider mental illness (Chapter 7) and abnormal parenting's effect on the architecture of the brain (hyper-vigilance, for example) and how mindfulness can be used to establish "ordinary parenting".
- consider disabilities (Chapter 8) and if parents could ever imagine their child in a wheelchair, blind, with profound learning disability, and growing into disabled adults totally dependent on others ... and how these babies self-regulate so that parents no longer feel they are being rejected.
- consider fathers (Chapter 9) – internalised or otherwise – and how they are entangled in the eyes and lives of mothers and infants and how mindfulness can "de-charge" parents to see their baby in a neutral and benevolent way.

And lastly, Dr Pozzi asks us to:

- consider breaking the cycle (Chapter 10) with the help of analysis (now parent-infant psychotherapy) whereas Klein describes, "a child begins to show stronger constructive tendencies, [...] changing relations to its father or mother, or to its brothers and sisters, [...] and a growth of social feeling" (Klein, 1933, p. 255).

Presented in a straight-forward style, these are the arguments Dr Pozzi asks us to consider. She is asking us to consider mindfulness as a "shortcut" to better results. Why? She tells us straight up: "to allow [parents] to see the baby as a separate being, as a little person with his or her own mind". This is her core objective. She tells us how to do this, given the forces set against us (these forces against us are her chapter titles: pregnancy, guilt, dislocation and loss, mental illness, and disabilities). These forces set up destructive cycles too strong to be broken ... or can they? Can we re-write what John Byng-Hall calls "family scripts"?

Dr Pozzi wants us to see therapy as an opportunity. And she argues that therapists have a commitment to continually offer better therapy. We must nudge our therapy into better outcomes without abandoning what we know and what experience has shown us to be effective. Over the years, therapy has become multi-disciplinary, more focused and intensive, and therapy now aims to reset the line of development in such a self-sustaining way that the client/family continues to improve even when the formal part of therapy is over. In parent-infant work, therapy becomes an intervention. In my own career focus on at-risk situations – in the books I've written, the clinic I've started (the first in the UK), the school I founded (also the first in the UK) and in the charity I founded – I've seen that the most effective interventions can never be too early. And the most effective way to intervene early is to work through relationships to reconnect the child with the family and vice-versa. This is the essence of parent-infant psychotherapy. Working through relationships is what distinguishes parent-infant psychotherapy from all of the other applied psychologies.

In this "writing project", Dr Pozzi shows us that mindfulness can be a useful element of a multi-disciplinary strategy. Although mindfulness is not easy to do – directing breath, observing baby, themselves and the stream of thoughts and feelings flowing through their mind – the practice of mindfulness provides a structural framework on which progress can be made:

- it is concise – allowing therapists access to the affective world of a child where they can be transformation agents.
- it connects – emotional experience to biological processes.
- it integrates – the rediscovery of ancient wisdom (head/heart), it can help to increase one's awareness of the destructive effects of one's addiction and that a possible relapse is transitory and not fixed for ever and ever.
- it is a guide ... DBT (Dialectic Behaviour Therapy), MBCT (Mindfulness-Based Cognitive Therapy) and Acceptance and Commitment Therapy (ACT) ... all of these derivative therapies help participants to become aware and to disengage by responding differently to their negative, ruminative thoughts and feelings that may propel them even further into depression.
- it fuses – bringing the multi-disciplinary work into a therapy unit.

Best of all,

- it is interesting.

Perhaps like me, you'll realise that this "writing project" has been written by someone at the top of her game, a perspective from the pinnacle. In no small sense, this is a biography of sorts, the author's professional life condensed to conclusions supported by a chain of logic stretching from the brain's inner workings to mountaintop transcendence. But in another sense, this is a guide for therapists – shorter than a handbook but not quite a map – which is useful in connecting-the-dots and navigating the interacting landscapes of neuro biology and development, mental health, early intervention and family wellness ... and the power of getting the therapy right.

I've always admired Maria Pozzi as a good therapist. This "writing project" is her latest offering showing she is an innovator and good thinker as well. She brings to her writing insight (e.g. she describes "real friends were her churning thoughts"), experience, and "solid tears". As an innovator, she brings mindfulness into the treatment space, as effective in dealing with our thoughts as transference and countertransference deal with our feelings and emotions.

Stella Acquarone, PhD

Reference

Klein, M. (1933). The early development of conscience in the child. In *Love, Guilt and Reparation* (pp. 248–257). London: The Hogarth Press, 1975.

Introduction

and of that second kingdom will I sing
wherein the human spirit doeth purge itself
and to ascend to Heaven
becometh worth.
                    Dante, Purgatory *vv. 4–6*

Some moments – perhaps rare – in the life of a baby, can be thought of as meditative moments. In the tranquil time when a baby has been cleaned, fed and rests embraced by his mother's loving lap and gaze; or when he – from his bouncy chair – looks around alert, not fretful, alone but not lonely, at those times we may think of him as being like a little Buddha. Yet, at many other times, such a blissful state is replaced by screams, demanding needs, uncomfortable states, stress and unhappiness that concern and unsettle the parents of this young and helpless creature. If sensitive and wise adults are part of this baby's environment, and if the unsettlement persists, a prompt referral to a local parent and baby service – although not yet enough of these are around the Country – can be made. In England there is an organisation named PIP-UK (Parent-Infant Partnership), which – together with the internationally renowned Anna Freud, Tavistock Centres and the Parent-Infant Clinic – provide psychotherapeutic interventions to distressed families with infants.

This book intends to explore – in the related chapters – the value, the complementarity and the changes produced in the growing infant, in his developing brain and in his family, by both parent-infant psychotherapy and mindfulness offered to families in distress. It explores at which point in a session mindfulness is introduced, is explained by the therapist, demonstrated and practiced there and then together with parents and babies.

The chosen topics refer mostly to the parental difficulties and mental states rather than to the baby's possible presenting symptoms, which may have not yet manifested themselves. This choice is dictated by the effect of the transformative work with the parents that allows babies to gain again central position in the parents' mind. This is in line with what we read in the recent Psychodynamic Diagnostic Manual (PDM2, 2017): "Mental development during infancy and early childhood reflects dynamic relationships among many dimensions of human functioning, including emotional, social, language, cognitive, regulatory-sensory processing, and motor capacities." (Ibid., p. 625). It affirms that infant experiences can only be understood within a relational, social and cultural context and, I would add, the infant can only grow healthily within a good relationship with a maternal or paternal figure. In the ongoing debate about the effect of "nature" and "nurture", there has been

> a greater emphasis on "nurture" – that is the postnatal family environment as the primary determinant of individual differences. [...] developmental biology and neuroscience tend to view development through a "nature" lens. [...] The emerging field of epigenetics offers the potential to unite these divergent perspectives in surprising and exciting ways.
>
> (Ibid., p. 505)

Epigenetics describes the interplay between genes and environment and indicates that chronic exposure to adversity shapes the physiological and behavioural development: experiential and biological influences are highly intertwined. A combination of several factors shapes the personality of the infant. "These include: (1) epigenetics, (2) temperament, (3) neuropsychology, (4) attachment style, (5) defensive style, (6) sociocultural factors." (Ibid., p. 504)

The choice of which parent-infant dyad or triad is most representative of one specific problem has been difficult due to the overlapping and co-morbidity of situations; for example, risk in pregnancy can be posed by diverse causes such as mental illness, alcoholism, previous losses etc. I will therefore choose the most extensive and severe family situation to be representative of that specific topic.

The term family will be preferred to describe any referred mother-baby or the triad, which includes fathers and siblings; fathers can be present in the mind of the mother and baby, even if not physically attending sessions. I will also use the term maternal to include any other primary carer performing a maternal function.

The male pronoun "he" will be used to define the baby in general terms and when not referred to a specific female baby.

Bibliography

Dante, A. The Divine Commedy: Purgatorio Canto I, vv 4–6.
Psychodynamic Diagnostic Manual, Second Edition PDM-2. (2017). Edited by Lingiardi, V. and McWilliams, N. New York: Guilford Press.

1 What is parent-infant psychotherapy?

Do you have the patience to wait
Till your mud settles and the water is clear?
Can you remain unmoving
Till the right action arises by itself?
                    Lao Tzu, 500 BC, p. 6

Parent-infant psychotherapy is a form of brief treatment that in the past decades has become very popular worldwide. It addresses families with infants and relies on the notion that this age group presents dramatic and intense psychological and emotional states, which have not become ossified and rigidified yet, and can be modified by interventions even of a short duration. Early interventions already have a therapeutic function as they can free infants and families on the path of development. They also perform a preventative function in addressing early anxieties and concerns in their budding and often contain and resolve them permanently. The work with infants raises very different concerns and problems from working with older children. The pressure put upon the worker is enormous, as the baby cannot wait for the parents to take time to change. There is an urgency in working with infants, which pressures us to find the promptest and best way of intervening. Several authors have pointed this out[1]:

Brazelton and Cramer (1991); Daws (1999); Hopkins (1994); Miller (1992); Pawl and Lieberman (1997). Morgan in her interview by Paul and Thomson-Salo (2001); Acquarone (2016); Baradon (2002); Baradon and Biseo (2016); Emanuel (2002); Lieberman and Van Horn (2008); Norman (2001); Paul and Thomson-Salo (2014); Pozzi-Monzo and Tydeman (2007); Salomonsson (2014). The infant cannot wait for the parents to sort out their long-standing problems, due to the pressure of the developmental phases ushering in.

Working with parents and babies, whether in the first or last session, relies greatly on the observation and understanding of the here and now. The therapist elicits an account of the problems, concern, symptomatic behaviour, the child's early history and the parents' own experiences in their families of origin. Also, the therapist sharpens his or her attention and observation of the nuances of the infant's expressions, movements and interactions with the parents. As it appears appropriate, the therapist can just listen silently or offer a descriptive commentary of the emotions, fears, worries, conflicts etc., which are expressed by the family members, or can make links with what is being recounted. Interest, curiosity and a capacity to observe are paramount in this work as in all psychological therapies.

Both the World and the UK Associations of Infant Mental Health (WAIMH and AIMH) and Parent Infant Partnership United Kingdom (PIP-UK) aim at bringing together professionals who are aware of the necessity for a good start in life and who would promote the psychological needs and mental welfare of infants and their parents. They provide information, publicity, study days and congresses to create links between clinicians and researchers.

The pioneers

Psychoanalysis – since Freud's times – has always recognised the importance and value of early years' foundation in the development of the personality. Freud himself came to understand some unconscious phantasies of children's, as he treated both Little Hans via his father, and also adult patients, whose severe psychopathology he could detect as being rooted in early childhood (Freud, 1909, 1918). His theoretical and clinical practice was imbued with awareness and many discoveries on infantile development of mental structure, sexuality, phantasy etc. (Freud, 1905, 1907, 1908, 1909, 1909b, 1918). The pioneers in child analysis Anna Freud (Freud, 1936, 1965) and Melanie Klein (Klein, 1926–1961) devoted their thinking, understanding and clinical work almost entirely to the early anxieties, conflicts, defences, phantasies and psychological functioning of children of all ages within their family context. They were also keenly interested in the child within the adult patient. They have opened up a huge field of discoveries and knowledge pertinent to the early years.

Winnicott

Donald W. Winnicott was the first clinician, who practised and wrote about a type of brief intervention with mothers seen together with their infants. His therapeutic interventions were not formally considered a treatment process; therefore, despite his work having inspired many clinicians, it was Selma Fraiberg, who was formally recognised as the founder of parent-infant psychotherapy. Winnicott was at great ease in talking to children and parents and was a skilled observer of the infant-mother dyad, which he saw as a psychic unit. He developed a unique way of assessing and treating symptoms linked with this dyad, and of assisting parents in the difficult task of rearing children (1941). The spatula technique permitted him to make a rapid diagnosis and treatment, as in the case of seven-month-old Margaret suffering from asthmatic wheezing. Winnicott used to place within reach of baby Margaret the spatula or tongue depressor within reach of the baby and observed her response. Margaret sat on her mother's lap while mother held her chest with her two hands supporting the baby's body and indicating the exaggerated movement of her chest.

> The asthma occurred on both occasions over the period in which the child hesitated about taking the spatula. She put her hand to the spatula and then, as she controlled her body, her hand and her environment, she developed asthma, [...] at the moment when she came to feel confident about the spatula which was at her mouth [...] the asthma ceased.
>
> (1941, p. 58)

It is interesting to read that after two consultations the baby no longer suffered from asthma but, Winnicott wrote that her mother became bronchially asthmatic. He thought that "the parent's attitude does make a lot of difference in certain cases [... although] generally speaking, the baby's normal hesitation cannot be explained by a reference to the parental attitude" (Ibid., p. 59). This happened in 1941 and we can see a form of parent-infant psychotherapy in embryo. Winnicott, who recognised the input of both the child and the parent in a problematic relationship, pioneered the idea of parental projection, which has more recently become a widely spread way of looking at some of children's psychological difficulties and of understanding parent-child relationships (Winnicott, 1941).

Selma Fraiberg

In 1975, in San Francisco, the Freudian psychoanalyst Selma Fraiberg and her team pioneered and formalised a method of treatment which was to become the Manifesto of parent-infant psychotherapy and pillar for further forms of parent-infant psychotherapy. In her seminal paper "Ghosts in the Nursery: A Psychoanalytic Approach to the Problems of Impaired Infant-Mother Relationship" (1975), she wrote that the experience with children in the present, is shadowed by the parents' unresolved past history of abuse and violence.

The affect, i.e. the emotional experience of such past events, had undergone repression and is not available to the parents, while they ill-treat their children. The parent repeats the past, "identifies with the aggressor of the past" (Fraiberg, 1975, p. 194) and acts it out with his or her baby/child in the present. Mrs March could never hear her five and a half-month-old baby's cries, as she was never heard as a baby by her mother, who had suffered from postpartum psychosis and abandoned her. The ghosts from her past inhabited the child's nursery. It is through the re-experience – in the present, therapeutic context – of the early anxieties, sufferings and feelings that the parent becomes emotionally reconnected with the affects of the original experience. The parent is freed of the repetition of the past and becomes able to identify with a protector figure and a loving parent for his or her child.

It is the relationship between parents and infants or toddlers, which is treated in this approach and even the youngest baby, is an eloquent participant in the dialogue in this therapy. The type of patients treated by the San Francisco Group can be categorised as difficult to reach and a modification of technique was necessary in order to achieve therapeutic results. Specific aspects of this model of intervention are that the therapy usually takes place in the family's home, as this is the family choice, hence the nickname of "psychotherapy in the kitchen". Concrete assistance is an important aspect of this programme as the material difficulties most of these families struggle with, represent real threats to parents and children and need addressing. Also, developmental guidance is offered as a way of normalising the child's experience, even in cases of behaviours, which radically deviate from the norm. Parents can be helped to support the child's developmental thrust, when they know what is to be expected of the child at that particular age.

Current thinkers

Abraham Brafman

Brafman (2001) in one of his books on working with children and parents grounds his practice as a child psychoanalyst in Winnicott's contribution and thinking. Brafman is not one of the best-known clinicians in the area of infant-parents psychotherapy, but it is worthwhile considering his approach. He writes about the three basic principles that guide his work, where the parents are intimately involved in the therapeutic interventions with their children. He writes:

> (1) our present is influenced by earlier experiences; (2) our behaviour and conscious life is influenced by our unconscious feelings and fantasies; and (3) child and parents influence each other in such a way that it may be impossible to establish what is cause and what is effect in their interactions.
>
> (Ibid., p. 2)

He emphasises that the parent-child relationship is affected by mutual influences or projections and it is hard to know what comes first and where the "knot" begins. Brafman refers to Winnicott's use of the word "knot" to indicate that the "child's presenting symptoms will [...] point to a possible obstacle that the parents cannot overcome because of some unconscious factor of their own" (Ibid., p. 27). The knot, he continues, "is also a useful description of a similar specific blockage in one or both parents' parenting functions. For the sake of brevity, we can say that the child and parents have become caught in a 'knot'" (Ibid. p. 27).

The concept of "knot" has some resonance in Fraiberg's idea of "ghosts in the nursery" (Fraiberg et al., 1975) and in my idea of a "hook" (Pozzi, 2003), which I learnt from the mother of a four-year-old girl during a family session when the child, "the parent, or both parents, are caught up with each other in a relationship that becomes like a tug-of-war and is far from being the container-contained relationship described by Bion" (Pozzi, 2003, p. 4).

Brafman uses the technical device of drawing, of closely observing child and mother together as well as the family history and the possible parental conflicts regarding the presenting problem in the child, as in the case of 13-month-old David, referred for indiscriminate biting (2001, p. 71). Brafman, in true Winnicottian style, has very much the child's conflicts and anxieties at the centre of his therapeutic consultations. He seems to pose himself as an observer of the child-parent dyad and is quite open in exploring his thinking processes and feelings with the dyad.

Paul Trad

Coming from a rather different approach and a medical model, Paul Trad in his book *Short-Term Parent-Infant Psychotherapy* (1993) relies on some traditional concepts from individual short-term work with patients. He actively challenges the patient's resistance and proactively proposes a "plan of action" which "requires the parent/patient to complete certain concrete assignments at each session" and "patient and therapist collaborate on a strategy for asserting goal-oriented outcomes" (Trad, 1993, p. 54). He does not pursue the connections with unresolved issues in the past but rather introduces a new technique, which he calls "previewing", to connect the mother, as main provider, to her infant. "Previewing" implies having distinct representations of the baby during pregnancy and also an anticipation of "upcoming developmental events for [her] infant in a dynamic fashion" (Ibid., p. 7). He works entirely with the mother-infant dyad and "teaches [mothers] how to engage in previewing behaviours with their infants" (Ibid., p. 153). He does not involve fathers, unlike many therapists and analysts from all over the globe and child psychotherapists in England tend to do (Barrows, 1999). Trad explicitly disavows the transference and countertransference, important clinical tools for other schools of parent-infant psychotherapy, such as the British School.

The Geneva School

The Geneva School outlines the clinical and technical bases for its model, which combines a child development and psychoanalytic approach and focuses on the parental representational world, projected onto the child. Its founders have published extensively on their way of working (Cramer, 1995, 2000; Palacio-Espasa, 1993; Stern, 1995, 1998). Here are some basic principles underlying this intervention model, which is mostly brief and based on a limited number of sessions offered to families.

This therapy model is based on the belief and clinical observation that both babies and their parents show great resilience, "self-correcting tendencies and energy for adaptation, which are probably stronger in this early period and in young parenthood than they will ever be again [... Therefore] infancy is an ideal period for brief intervention" (Brazelton and Cramer, 1991, pp. 173–4).

The time after the birth of a child is particularly charged psychologically, especially for first-time parents. It is a time of crisis since the usual defensive strategies employed by parents, mothers in particular, have to be re-organised and a new parental identity has to be found. Parents are more vulnerable to conflicts but also more resilient, receptive to the surrounding environment, open to new learning, to changes and this favours their availability to use psychotherapy (Brazelton and Cramer, 1991; Palacio-Espasa, 1993).

The disturbances treated are commonly functional and behavioural symptoms in the infant: sleep and feeding disorders, crying, agitation, bonding etc. ...

It is well known that very intense anxieties are felt by mothers regarding the possible death of their baby. The extreme dependency and vulnerability of the infant seem to stir up deep death anguish, which can push some mothers to remove themselves from being close to the baby.

The Geneva thinkers reckon that to offer support to parents and insight into their projections, anxieties and ambivalence at this point in their life, releases positive forces for attachment so that growth and normal maturational processes can resume. The mother and the baby in their very different modes of functioning, easily intermesh with their psychic functioning with mutual projections and representations, during the first 18 months of the baby's life. They both become highly motivated "partners" in the therapeutic adventure. A mother's transparency of thoughts, feelings and fantasies about her baby is somehow demonstrated by the infant, who usually behaves and illustrates the maternal scenarios, pointing at the failing interaction, during sessions.

This requires "dual attention" from the therapist, who listens carefully to the mother's accounts and watches the baby's behaviour and reaction and their mutual interacting.

Usually between one and ten sessions are needed to bring about considerable changes and the mother-infant couple is seen at a weekly interval for an hour.

The therapist's interventions aim mainly at unfolding maternal anxieties and projections of old ghosts, (Fraiberg et al., 1975), which distort her capacity to see the baby more objectively and to link those with the infant's symptom. This constitutes the "focus" (Malan, 1976) or "core conflictual relationship theme" (Luborsky, 1990) of this brief mother-infant therapy. The child's symptom is understood as a reaction to maternal impingement and it provides the mother some defences against her own anxiety, guilt and depression. The therapy aims at interpreting the emerged focus and modifying the underlying anxieties and conflicts in the mother, in order to allow a new relationship to evolve.

The Geneva therapists do not make transference interpretations about the mother's transference to the therapist and their main focus is the mother's transference to her infant. Also, they do not state how transference and countertransference inform their working model.

Fathers, who may also attend these sessions, are indeed thought of as very important, as Brazelton and Cramer wrote explicitly in a chapter in *The Earliest Relationship* (1991). However, fathers do not figure much in the work described by these clinicians, even though they are apparently indirectly affected and their representations of the child change during the work with the mother-infant dyad (Cramer et al., 1990). In a recent paper Palacio-Espasa (2004) writes that the father's contribution can be quite similar to the mother's and that the representations of both parents have to be worked on in this brief therapy. He also noticed through his clinical practice, that the success of brief triadic psychotherapeutic interventions seems to rely on a well-balanced relationship in the couple.

The Geneva group with Cramer et al. (1990), Robert-Tissot et al. (1996, 1999, 2004) and their team have produced – in the past 25 years – systematic outcome studies on evaluation, effectiveness, comparison of different psychotherapies, patients' choice of treatment etc., to mention a few. They remain aware of the difficulties in assessing outcome and process in psychotherapy. However, clinicians and researchers on that team, have worked together in an impressive way to keep a marriage going by mutual and acceptable compromises, which do not interfere with searching for truth and understanding beyond individual ideologies, as Cramer eloquently put it (Cramer, 2000).

Due to ethical concerns regarding the problem of having a control group in their research, the Geneva clinicians opted for an alternative type of brief intervention called Interactional Guidance, originally designed by Susan McDonough (1992) in the United States, to help multi-problem families not amenable to verbal-type therapies. The mother's play with her child is videotaped during sessions and later shown and discussed with her. The therapist reinforces positive features and supports parental competencies.

A very detailed analysis of these two therapies, their differences and similarities in focus, technique, processes, symptoms, changes in maternal representations, measures, assessment tools, results etc., is written about in several papers (Cramer, 1998; Cramer et al., 1990; Robert-Tissot et al., 1996).

An interesting outcome is that both forms of therapy are effective in: producing changes in functional and behavioural symptoms in the child (sleep and eating disorders, crying, agitation, aggression); in changing maternal representations of the child; in increasing maternal self-esteem and lowering maternal depression. These changes applied differently to the two types of therapy but were maintained at six months post-test evaluation in both cases.

Palacio-Espasa and Juan Manzano, who also work with the Geneva group, think of themselves as being influenced by Freud, Klein and Bion more than their other colleagues Cramer, Stern and Brazelton, who rely a lot more on developmental concepts and attachment theory. Palacio-Espasa and Manzano focus mainly on clinical work and attempt to conceptualise and classify theoretical and technical aspects of parent-infant psychotherapy. They formulate their theoretical and technical ideas beautifully and extensively, with regard to the type of parental conflict, of projections on the child, of pre-transference to the therapist and to the child's Oedipal or pre-Oedipal conflicts and psychopathology.

In their thinking, they use Freudian and Kleinian concepts, models of the mind and language, and this resembles, in part, the work of many child psychotherapists as well as that of some other clinicians engaged in parent-infant psychotherapy. Here are some of their original ideas.

It is the mother-child and occasionally the father-child relationship and the nature of their bond or link, which manifests a psychopathological aspect, such as a possible symbiotic, rejecting or intrusive link between mother/main carer and child. This type of link or relationship becomes the object of therapeutic interventions in these authors' brief treatments. The authors share the general view that such treatments can affect and resolve the symptoms in the child but also bring about structural changes in the parental pathology and ultimately in the parent-child conflicts.

The birth of a new baby, especially the first one, changes the couple's identity, which is now faced with the task of becoming parents. The young adult has to take care of the new baby and this requires identification with one's parents or parental figures. Old unresolved conflicts can be re-activated and the new-born can become the vessel of the parents' infantile, unresolved conflicts and vindication. The authors call this new conflictual state "conflictuality of parenthood" (Manzano et al., 1999). In this scenario, the baby can be invested by a variety of parental desires, ideals and expectations and can be perceived as a dangerous id, dominated by needs and instinctual demands, or as a super-ego, critical and authoritarian in its demands. The "conflictuality of parenthood" takes on a specific quality, defined by the authors "narcissistic parental conflictuality", since the parent tends to represent him or herself in this process of projective identification with the child.

The word narcissistic is intended as both "self-love" and as: "an object-type representation of the other that has become the subject's own self through fantasies of introjective and projective identification that may wholly or partially obliterate the boundaries between self and object" (Manzano et al., 1999, p. 469). This means that parents project their own parts, wishes or ideas into their child as well as identify with him, in a way that is parent-focused i.e. narcissistically centred. This easily leads to blur the difference between the parent and the child and to prevent separateness.

However, the authors believe that: "... in the context of parent-child relations the notion of projective identification does not necessarily have a pathological connotation. Projective identification with a child may be a vehicle for parental empathy with him and thereby contribute to his psychic development" (Ibid., p. 468). They also notice that it is part of ordinary parenthood to project on one's child but also to be able to see the child in his or her own right. In London, child psychotherapist Likierman also reckons that maternal love and positive projective identification are part of ordinary child development and internalisation of good objects (Likierman, 1988).

The above-mentioned authors from the Geneva School explore a typology of unconscious phantasies that a parent can project on the new-born and live out accordingly. A first group of unconscious phantasies is about parental past losses, which have not been properly mourned. The birth of the baby awakens a new hope in the parent to deny that old, unresolved loss. It can be a real loss of a dear person or of an ideal object or a phantasy. Another parent may project the wished-for ideal baby that the parent would have liked to have been and may identify with the wished-for ideal parent. In this way, there is an attempt to resolve an old conflictual situation. In another scenario, the parent projects the memory of the loved child the parent had once been and identifies with his/her good parents of the past. In this way, a separation from the past has not taken place. These types of projected, unconscious phantasies border with normality but can become pathological depending on their intensity, violent, aggressive or omnipotent quality or when they are used defensively by the parent in order to deny separation anxieties and object-loss.

As well as these pre-Oedipal phantasies, also Oedipal ones of exclusion, jealousy and rivalry belong to this "libidinal constellation", as the authors call it. This implies that the main aim achieved by this type of projections is for the parent to regain a lost object, which was never properly mourned. When these projected phantasies persist, the parent has a positive investment on the child and a positive pre-transference to the therapist. This kind of organisation is called by the authors "neurotic or depressive conflictuality" and it offers a good prognosis and successful outcome in brief parent-child psychotherapy.

Another group of unconscious phantasies projected on the child belongs to a more pathological, parental constellation. The child is seen as a vessel of expelled parental, internal objects or parts of the self, which are persecutory and unwanted. The child becomes an object of hatred and aggression and is projectively identified with the maltreated child of the parent's past. The parent, in turn, is identified with the maltreating and abusive parent of the past. The actual parent may also react and overcompensate for a harsh, strict or rejecting experience with the parent of the past, by overindulging and intruding the present child.

These projections represent parental, paranoid-schizoid states of mind, described as "narcissistic conflictuality" and usually require long-term, individual intervention for the parent. The parental pre-transference to the therapist is also characterised by hostile and negative feelings and this renders short-term psychotherapy very difficult or virtually impossible, according to the authors. The interpreted parent-child transference and the non-interpreted positive pre-transference to the therapist are seen as contributing to changes in these treatments.

Another element that fosters changes is the parent's state of need and moment of crisis, which increase the availability, the emotional mobility and the reparatory wish in the parent. Also, the infant's open and not-yet-fixed psychic organisation is particularly receptive to the therapist's early intervention. The therapist's attention to the infant's play and communication, to the parent's unconscious phantasies and their interpretation to both parent and baby, facilitate a resolution of the parent-infant conflicts, which are overtly external-ised in their interactions and play.

All this is rather different from the other clinicians of the Geneva Group and I, indeed, think that transference and countertransference are essential tools in this work.

The baby at the centre of treatment

As we have seen so far, an essential aspect of parent-infant, or infant-parent psychotherapy as some authors prefer to call it, is the presence of the baby, who together with the parents, stage the conflict in the here and now of the ses-sion, thus allowing the therapist to observe and understand such conflict and to verbalise the underlying links with the symptomatic behaviour.

Norman, Salomonsson and Morgan present a different focus in their infant-parent working model from the authors so far quoted. They believe in the importance and necessity to actively work with the infant and to make a verbal link between the analyst and the infant, seen as an individual in his or her own right. This will not take away anything from the intimate relationship between mother and infant but will offer the infant a new experience of containment (Norman, 2001) and the mother a gap or transitional space, which will allow growth to both mother, father and infant, as Morgan recounted in her interview with Frances Salo (Thomson Salo, 2001).

Johan Norman and Bjorn Salomonsson in Sweden

Norman, a Swedish psychoanalyst reflected on the idea that Fraiberg and the clinicians from the Geneva School focused on the parental representation of the infant and the effect such representation had on the parent-infant relationship. This was their target of understanding and change and not the infant himself: their main therapeutic relationship was with the parents, not with the infant.

Norman (2001, 2004) worked intensively and long-term – when needed – with the infant and the mother, but focused on the infant by describing detailed visual and vocal expressions and movements produced by the infant in response to the analyst talking to him. For example, he introduced himself to 20-month-old baby Tim, born at 25 weeks' gestation, in their first encounter and soon after mother had mentioned Tim's anxiety about their meeting (Norman, 2001).

> Tim looked at me, apparently wondering. I turned my attention to him, saying,
> "My name is Johan. We don't know each other yet, but your mother has asked me to meet with you and her to see if I can help you both." He gave a sudden, wry smile, rather a grimace of fear and rejection, and bared his white teeth like a cornered animal. I said, "I realise that you are frightened".
>
> (Ibid., p. 86)

Norman's innovative way of working with troubled infants and their parents is by creating a strong emotional link with the non-verbal infant by talking to him and by creating a transference between the infant and the analyst in the analytic setting. In this way a containing link is restored between the infant and the mother, too. Repressed and inhibited feelings of hatred and aggression find expression in the analytic setting, which had previously manifested themselves in the form of aversion reactions towards the mother and in the infant's sudden and prolonged whining. The analyst, by offering reverie and containment of the infant and mother, as a

> third object not involved in the disturbance [...] may reactivate and retrieve those parts of the infant's inner world that have been excluded from containment, leading to a vitalisation of the emotional disturbance that can then be worked through in the mother-infant relationship.
>
> (Norman, 2001, p. 97)

This provides mother and infant with a reparatory experience and hope. Norman reckons that Meltzer's distinction (Meltzer, 1986 cited in Norman, 2001) between the lexical meaning of the word and the non-lexical aspect of it, is rather useful to build a picture of what level of comprehension can be established with the infant.

> The non-lexical aspect is the affective language expressed in gestures, facial expressions, the music of the voice and the body language. The meaning of the message will be expressed simultaneously in these different languages, the lexical and the non-lexical. [... there] is reason to assume that infants, long before they can talk, have a comprehension of the non-lexical, affective language.
>
> (Norman, 2001, p. 84)

Salomonsson (2014) follows very much in his teacher's footsteps in talking with infants in the presence of their parents but he adds a research component to his work. A Randomised Controlled Trial (RCT) of MIP (Mother Infant Psychoanalytic) treatment was carried out using different instruments to evaluate the efficacy of this treatment. It showed a decrease in maternal depression and stress, increased sensitivity and quality of dyadic relationships and consequently calmer and more settled babies.

Ann Morgan, Campbell Paul and Frances Thomson-Salo in Australia

These authors at the Royal Children's hospital in Melbourne shared Norman's view that the baby is a subject in his or her own right and therefore, active work with the infant is a "must." Not "seeing" and not working with the infant is a way of colluding with the parental hatred and murderous phantasies towards the infant. If such negative feelings are not faced, even by the therapist, the intergenerational transmission of difficulties will continue (Paul and Thomson-Salo, 2001). These authors had a wide range of experience in seeing severely disturbed infants. They are well aware that, while mothers recover from their illnesses, the situation is urgent for the infant, psychologically as well as in terms of physical development (including brain functioning and development) which set in fast and are tightly linked with the experience of attachment. In relating directly to the infant, they offer an experience of connection with such infants, aiming at creating a gap between mother and infant, a sort of transitional space in which they work with both the parents' toxic and hateful projections onto the infant and with the infant, who can then be seen by the mother in a new light. They also stressed that it is the parental couple, which is more relevant to the infant's development, rather than the mother with her own mother as Stern had postulated (1995).

Amongst many other authors who have taken an interest in parent-infant psychotherapy, I would like to mention Berg in South Africa, Watillon in Brussels, Pawl & Lieberman in New York and Blos Jr. in Philadelphia.

Astrid Berg and issues of cultural diversity

Astrid Berg works in a community well-baby clinic in a slum area outside Cape Town and brings to our attention the interesting and broader perspective of parent-infant psychotherapy, seen in its cultural context. She uses the model of parental representation as a focal point to achieve changes in parent-infant psychotherapy, but expands it to the traditional African social fabric and its pivotal attitude of reverence for the ancestors. She explains the universal, African belief that something of the dead person does not wholly disappear but survives in the living and will act as an inner guide. This is somewhat in line with Freud's notion of the work of mourning (Freud, 1917). However, in this cultural view, the ancestors have to be taken care of, for them to act as guides and mentors of the living, otherwise they will withdraw their protection and expose the individual or family to the evil of witchcraft. The nuclear family is contained within the clan, which is in turn connected to the ancestors. Berg writes of a tragic case, where a mother and her baby "were left without the protective blanket of tradition and culture", since the mother had to turn to prostitution because of poverty, became pregnant and lost her place with her husband and the clan. This led to the removal of her by-then-autistic baby. What was missing in the handling of this mother and baby, writes Berg, was a full awareness of the level of this couple's isolation from their culture and cruel consequences of it (Berg, 2000).

Annette Watillon in Belgium

Watillon considers two subgroups of parent-infant psychotherapy, depending on whether the referred child is an infant or older than two and she adapts her technique accordingly. Transference interpretations are made to the child in the presence of the parents who will gain a better understanding of the fundamental place of the child's psychic reality and will be able retrospectively to make sense of certain forms of behaviour which they experience as strange or even as pathological. In this way, too, they will gain access to the affective world of a child ...

(Watillon, 1993, p. 1042)

She stresses one factor, which accounts for the mutative effect of these consultations, i.e. the dramatisation and externalisation of the relational conflict of the participants in the sessions, similarly to certain aspects of psychodrama (Ibid., p. 1041). She continues that the analyst, by acting both as a theatre director and as a fellow-actor in the performance at different times, fulfils a transforming function in the scenario. Watillon reckons that with children over two, the length of treatment has to be adjusted to obtain results in a few sessions.

Jeree Pawl and Alicia Lieberman in USA

Pawl & Lieberman share the general view that the hallmark of infant-parent psychotherapy is the infant's presence during treatment. However, they also see this as a possible interference in those situations where, for example, a parent may need to explore difficult, personal experiences but is constantly distracted by the child's demands. Therefore, they envisage a format where the child is absent from the session but firmly present in the therapist's mind (Pawl and Lieberman, 1997). They stress the paramount and mutative function of the qualities of the relationship between therapist and parent (Ibid., p. 342) and somehow privilege the parental component i.e. the parent-centred model rather than an infant-centred model of treatment. They embrace Fraiberg's model of providing concrete and practical support as well as emotional support, guidance and psychotherapy, depending on the parent's needs and requests. They deal with parents who have suffered from extreme neglect, deprivation and abuse as children, present antisocial personality and have negative expectations of services as well as a negative transference to the therapist. Therefore the

therapist needs to be conversant in normal and deviant development in infancy and toddlerhood as well as being skilled in assessing adult psychopathology and in clinical observation and intervention. As a result, the need for expertise in several areas, infant-parent psychotherapy is essentially a multidisciplinary undertaking.

(Ibid., p. 350)

Lieberman et al. (2015) in their more recent manual of parent-infant psychotherapy introduce the research component in their evidence-based treatment of traumatised and high-risk children and families. Multiple randomised control trials demonstrate the efficacy of their multidisciplinary approach in promoting quality of attachment and decreasing stress and traumas to children and families.

Peter Blos in USA

Peter Blos Jr. proposes a mother-centred approach to the treatment of mother-infant pairs. He focuses on the "unfinished developmental work of the mother which [he considers] to be a counterpoint to the infant and toddler separation-individuation" (Blos, 1985, p. 51). He writes that becoming a mother "brings up maternal identifications and, in part, rekindles the individuation issues of the past" (Ibid., p. 54). Therefore, due to the flexibility and the loosening of the defences in the maternal psychic structure of the after-birth period and up to about the eighteenth month of the child's life, there is an opportunity to re-work unfinished psychological individuation from primary objects. It is now the infant – no longer the mother's mother – who is experienced as the problem and as the malevolent agent. His is mostly a mother-centred model and there is no inclusion of the father in the therapeutic work.

The British schools

The Tavistock model

To return to the British scene and to the thinking and practice of parent-infant psychotherapy, there has been a broad proliferation of work, activities and papers in recent years.

The Tavistock model of working psycho-dynamically with small children and their families, has been known as Under-Five's Counselling – now called The Parent-Infant Mental Health Service – and has been practised, written about and researched extensively by Barrows (1999, 2000, 2004); Daws (1999); Emanuel (2002); Emanuel and Bradley (2008); Hopkins (1992, 1994); Likierman (1988); Miller (1992, 1994, 2000); Pozzi (2003); Pozzi and Tydeman (2005, 2007, 2011). This model originated in the mid-eighties under the leadership of Lisa Miller and Alan Shuttleworth and aimed at reaching promptly, those anxious parents who had become caught up in worries and stuck with the behaviour of their infants or young children. The philosophy of this approach is common to many other thinkers and recognises that, in becoming a parent, one's own past childhood experiences and unresolved conflicts can become re-activated and projected or re-enacted with one's own child. Plasticity is an aspect of both the early years and early parenthood and parents of infants and small children are particularly open and available to changes. This is a time when passions and turbulence are a daily experience and parents can easily feel overwhelmed by the intensity of the anxieties and symptoms presented by their infants and small children. Five sessions are usually offered to the whole family, although therapists work with whatever combination of family members come to the counselling.

Thinking about the presenting problem, how it came to be there in the first instance and how it affects family life etc. is one aim of this work.

The Infant Observation, as described by Esther Bick (Bick, 1964; Briggs, 2002; Sternberg, 2005), is an essential tool as it develops the observer's capacity to observe the family's scenarios and one's own emotional response as well as the capacity to begin to make space in one's mind for thinking and linking without judgement, action or precipitous interpretations. It also fosters the capacity for simultaneous identifications – what Bion called "binocular vision" and "multiple vertices" (Bion, 1965) – with the different people present during the observation or the counselling session and also with the many generations present in the participants' minds.

The therapist aims at understanding the emotions and phantasies felt and projected by the parent and related to the parent's unresolved ghosts (Fraiberg et al., 1975). To contain parental worries and anxieties and to comment in a way that helps the re-introjection of projections, define the success of this work. The therapist relies on the understanding of transference and countertransference for a more complete picture of what goes on in the here and now of these sessions, which is usually linked with the original problem. In this brief work, both the infant and the adult parent are the patients and it is with them both that the therapist tries to establish a dialogue that reaches their deep, unconscious hooks and helps them both to become unhooked (Pozzi, 2003).

The Anna Freud Centre

Since 2000, the team at the Anna Freud Centre have produced two versions of the book: *The Practice of Parent-Infant Psychotherapy: Claiming the Baby* (Baradon et al., 2005; Baradon and Biseo, 2016). The baby, born with a predisposition to relate, is at the centre of the psychoanalytic parent-infant psychotherapy and it is from this perspective that the book is written: the baby in relation to his primary carer and the baby's communicative way, which is non-verbal, behavioural, body-based and directed at the "other".

The following is taken from a review of the book (Pozzi, 2017):

> By observing the whole verbal and non-verbal presentation, by listening to the parent/s' concern, by engaging each family member, by modelling a new way of being together, by keeping the boundaries and being well aware of the countertransference, the therapist sets the scene either to offer or not to offer parent-infant psychotherapy. Cultural issues are accounted for sensitively and non-judgementally.
>
> (Ibid., pp. 296–7)

The early care-giving experiences "have a vital and life-long influence on the child's emotional, social and cognitive development. Genetic research has now demonstrated the impact of both the environment and the quality of attachment that can mitigate genetic influences. Equally the exposure to trauma and violence affects the baby's developing brain adversely. The baby's evolving sense of self develops by complete dependency on a human person and his earliest experiences become encoded in the procedural (unconscious) memory as 'body memory' (Ibid., p. 12). When adults become parents, they bring their own conscious and unconscious memories of having been parented into their relationship with their baby, whether good, abusive or traumatic: the ghosts and the angels in the nursery (Fraiberg et al., 1975; Lieberman et al., 2015). The baby's temperament and earliest experiences since his time in the womb also colour and impact the relationship with his parents, facilitating good enough care or reinforcing parental fragilities and psychological imbalances." The therapist acts as a new object for the baby, that is, engages physically with him in an embodied communication, for example, by stroking the infant's torso in rhythm with her voice. The transference relationship to the therapist – both negative and benevolent – is now recognised and verbalised and this fosters the link between the mother and her infant. The baby's transference to the therapist is also addressed directly with the baby, for example, "you're careful with me as you're afraid I will disappear and not come back like [your Dad]" (Baradon et al., 2016, p. 40). The use and value of filming the therapy (Woodhead et al., 2006) and ministering the Adult Attachment Interview (George et al., 1985) are important therapeutic tools to be employed in this work.

The Parent-Infant Clinic

The Parent-Infant Clinic was founded and is directed by Stella Acquarone since 1990 and has seen an innumerable number of babies and parents, who are struggling with issues such as bonding and attachment, post-natal depression, feeding, sleeping difficulties, excessive crying, failure to thrive and developmental delays. A multidisciplinary team of professionals work at the Clinic offering a variety of approaches: from observation of infants within their home environment or nursery, to psychological guidance to parents, psychoanalytic parent-infant psychotherapy, infant psychiatry and neuroscientific research. The Clinic has a particular take on autism and autistic spectrum disorders and offers intensive four-to-five week-long child-and-family treatments, which can penetrate the shell of autism, make sense of it and draw the child out and into being "an ordinary, little child" as one of the parents described the outcome of the therapeutic intervention received at the Clinic. As well as the clinic, Acquarone has also created a School of Infant Mental Health, which offers a four-year-long training to professionals working with infants and parents needing guidance, understanding and clinical interventions for their suffering infants, for their sense of hopelessness and for the involved-but-bewildered professionals.

As one can see from this excursus into the literature on parent-infant psychotherapy, many ideas and techniques flow together in a complementary, yet differentiated fashion. Some of these ideas will be explored and expanded in this book and will hopefully contribute to increase our understanding of the mysterious processes of psychotherapy.

Note

1 This chapter is based on a number of publications including my doctoral dissertation.

Bibliography

Acquarone, S. (2014). *Parent-Infant Psychotherapy: A Handbook*. London: Karnac Books.

Acquarone, S. (2016). *Changing Destinies*. London: Karnac Books.

Baradon, T. (2002). Psychotherapeutic Work with Parents and Infants – Psychodynamic and Attachment Perspectives. *Attachment and Human Development*, Vol. 4(1): 25–38.

Baradon, T. et al. (2005). *The Practice of Psychoanalytic Parent-Infant Psychotherapy*. London: Routledge.

Baradon, T., and Biseo, M. (2016). *The Practice of Psychoanalytic Parent-Infant Psychotherapy*. London and New York: Routledge.

Barrows, P. (1999). Fathers in Parent-Infant Psychotherapy. *Infant Mental Health Journal*, Vol. 20: 333–345.

Barrows, P. (2000). Making the Case for a Dedicated Infant Mental Health Service. *Psychoanalytic Psychotherapy*, Vol. 24(2): 111–128.

Barrows, P. (2004). Fathers and Families: Locating the Ghost in the Nursery. *Infant Mental Health Journal*, Vol. 25(5): 408–423.

Berg, A. (2000). Beyond the Dyad: Parent-Infant Psychotherapy in a Multi-Cultural Society. Reflection from a South African Perspective. Paper read at the 7th Congress of the W.A.I.M.H. – July, 2000. Montreal.

Bick, E. (1964). Notes on Infant Observation in Psychoanalytic Training. *The International Journal of Psychoanalysis*, Vol. 45: 558–566.

Bion, W.R. (1965). *Transformations*. London: Maresfield Reprints 1984, p. 145.

Bion, W.R. (1967). *Second Thoughts*. London: Maresfield Reprints.

Blos, P., Jr. (1985). Intergenerational Separation-Individuation. Treating the Mother-Infant Pair. *The Psychoanalytic Study of the Child*, Vol. 40: 41–56.

Brafman, A.H. (2001). *Untying the Knot: Working with Children and Parents*. London and New York: Karnac Books.

Brazelton, T.B., and Cramer, B.G. (1991). *The Earliest Relationship*. London: Karnac Books.

Briggs, A. (2002). *Surviving Space*. London: Karnac Books.

Cramer, B. (1995). Short-Term Dynamic Psychotherapy for Infants and Their Parents. *Child and Adolescent Psychiatric Clinics of North America*, Vol. 4: 649–659.

Cramer, B. (1998). Mother-Infant Psychotherapy: A Widening Scope in Technique. *Infant Mental Health Journal*, Vol. 19(2): 151–167.

Cramer, B. (2000). Bridging the Gap between Clinicians and Researchers. In: *W.A.I.M.H. Handbook of Infant Mental Health. Vol II*, pp. 271–312. Edited by Osofsky, J.D., Fitzgerald, H.E. New York: Wiley.

Cramer, B., Robert-Tissot, C., Stern, D.N., Serpa-Rusconi, S., De Muralt, M., Besson, G., Palacio-Espasa, F., Bachman, J.P., Knauer, D., Berney, C., and D'Arcys, U. (1990). Outcome Evaluation in Brief Mother-Infant Psychotherapy: A Preliminary Report. *Infant Mental Health Journal*, Vol. 11(3): 278–300.

Czogalik, D., and Mauthe, C. (1991). *Manual for the Stuttgart Interactional Categories System*. Research Report No 10. Stuttgart: Centre for Psychotherapy Research.

Daws, D. (1999). Brief Psychotherapy with Infant and Their Parents. In: *The Handbook of Child and Adolescent Psychotherapy*, pp. 261–272. Edited by Laniado, M., and Horne, A. London: Routledge.

Emanuel, L. (2002). Parents United: Addressing Parental Issues in Work with Infants and Young Children. *Infant Observation*, Vol. 5(2): 103–117.

Emanuel, L., and Bradley, E. (2008). *What Can the Matter Be?* London: Karnac Books.

Fraiberg, S., Adelson, E., and Shapiro, V. (1975). Ghosts in the Nursery. *Journal of the American Academy of Child Psychiatry*, Vol. 14: 387–421.

Freud, A. (1936). *The Ego and the Mechanisms of Defence*. London: Hogarth Press and The Institute of Psycho-Analysis.

Freud, A. (1965). *Normality and Pathology in Children*. New York: International Universities Press.

Freud, S. (1905). *Three Essays on the Theory of Sexuality*. S.E. Vol. 7: 123–245. London: The Hogarth Press.

Freud, S. (1907). *The Sexual Enlightenment of Children*. S.E. Vol. 9: 131. London: The Hogarth Press.

Freud, S. (1908). *On the Sexual Theories of Children*. S.E. Vol. 9: 209–226. London: The Hogarth Press.

Freud, S. (1909). *Analysis of a Phobia in a Five-Year-Old Boy*. S.E. Vol. 10: 5–149. London: The Hogarth Press.

Freud, S. (1909b). *Notes Upon a Case of Obsessional Neurosis*. S.E. Vol. 10: 155–318. London: The Hogarth Press.

Freud, S. (1917) *Mourning and Melancholia*. S.E. Vol. 14: 243–260. London: The Hogarth Press.

Freud, S. (1918). *From the History of an Infantile Neurosis*. S.E. Vol. 17: 9–123. London: The Hogarth Press.

George, C., Kaplan, N., and Main, M. (1985). *Adult Attachment Interview* (2nd ed.). Unpublished manuscript. Berkeley, CA: University of California.

Hopkins, J. (1992). Infant-Parent Psychotherapy. *Journal of Child Psychotherapy*, Vol. 18(1): 5–17.

Hopkins, J. (1994). Therapeutic Interventions in Infancy: Two Contrasting Cases of Persisting Crying. *Psychoanalytic Psychotherapy*, Vol. 8: 141–152.

Klein, M. (1926–1961). *The Writings of Melanie Klein*. Vol. 1–4. London: The Hogarth Press and The Institute of Psycho-Analysis.

Lieberman, A., Ghosh Ippen, C., and Van Horn, P. (2015). *Don't Hit My Mommy* (2nd ed.). Washington, DC: Zero to Three.

Lieberman, A.F., and Van Horn, P. (2008). *Psychotherapy with Infants and Young Children*. New York: The Guilford Press.

Likierman, M. (1988). Maternal Love and Positive Projective Identification. *Journal of Child Psychotherapy*, Vol. 14(2): 29–46.

Luborsky, L. (1990). A Guide to CCRT Method. In: *Understanding Transference: The CCRT Method*, pp. 15–36. Edited by Luborsky, L., and Crits-Christoph, P. New York: Basic Books.

Malan, D.H. (1976). *The Frontier of Brief Psychotherapy*. New York: Plenum.

Manzano, J., Palacio-Espasa, F., and Zilkha, N. (1999). The Narcissistic Scenario of Parenthood. *International Journal of Psychoanalysis*, Vol. 80: 465–476.

McDonough, S.C. (1992). L'aiuto All'interazione: Una Tecnica per Il Trattamento Dei Disturbi Relazionali Precoci. In: *Dalle Cure Materne All'interpretazione: Nuove Terapie per Il Bambino E Le Sue Relazioni: I Clinici Raccontano*, pp. 221–233. Edited by Fava Viziello, G., and Stern, D.N. Milano: Cortina.

Meltzer, D. (1986). *Studies in Extended Metapsychology: Clinical Applications of Boon's Ideas*. Perth: Clunie Press.

Miller, L. (1992). The Relation of Infant Observation to Clinical Practice in an under Fives Counselling Service. *Journal of Child Psychotherapy*, Vol. 18(1): 19–32.

Miller, L. (1994). Reviews. *Journal of Child Psychotherapy*, Vol. 20(3): 391–393. London: Routledge.

Miller, L. (2000). An under Five's Counselling Service and Its Relation to Questions of Assessment. In: *Assessment in Child Psychotherapy*, pp. 108–119. Edited by Rustin, M. and Quagliata, E. London: Duckworth.

Norman, J. (2001). The Psychoanalyst and the Baby: A New Look at Work with Infants. *International Journal of Psychoanalysis*, Vol. 82: 83–100.

Norman, J. (2004). Transformation of Early Infantile Experiences: A 6-Month-old-in Psychoanalysis. *International Journal of Psychoanalysis*, Vol. 85: 1103–1122.

Palacio-Espasa, F. (1993). La pratique psychothérapique avec l'enfant. In: *Italian: Psicoterapia con i bambini* (Bayard ed.). 1995, pp. 95–142. Milano: Cortina.

Palacio-Espasa, F. (2004). Parent-Infant Psychotherapy, the Transition to Parenthood and Parental Narcissism: Implications for Treatment. *Journal of Child Psychotherapy*, Vol. 30(2): 155–171.

Paul, C., and Thomson-Salo, F. (2014). *The Baby as Subject*. London: Karmac Books.

Pawl, J.H., and Lieberman, A.F. (1997). Infant-Parent Psychotherapy. In: *Handbook of Child and Adolescent Psychiatry*, Vol. 2, pp. 339–351. Edited by Noshpitz, J.D. New York: John Wiley Sons, Inc.

Pozzi, M. (2003). *Psychic Hooks and Bolts: Psychoanalytic Work with Children under Five and Their Families*. London and New York: Karnac Books.

Pozzi, M. (2017). Review of: The Practice of Psychoanalytic Parent–Infant Psychotherapy. Claiming the Baby, by Tessa Baradon and Michela Biseo, Oxford: Routledge. *Journal of Child Psychotherapy*, Vol. 43(2): 295–299.

Pozzi, M., and Tydeman, B. (2005). Setting Up a Counselling Service for Parents, Infants and Young Children. *Psychoanalytic Psychotherapy*, Vol. 19(4): 294–309.

Pozzi-Monzo, M., Lee, A., and Likierman, M. (2011). From Reactive to Reflective: Evidence for Shifts in Parents' State of Mind during Brief Under-fives Psychoanalytic Psychotherapy. *Clinical Child Psychology and Psychiatry*, Vol. 17(1): 151–164.

Pozzi-Monzo, M., and Tydeman, B. (2007). *Innovations in Parent-Infant Psychotherapy*. London: Karnac Books.

Robert-Tissot, C., and Cramer, B. (1998). When Patients Contribute to the Choice of Treatment. *Infant Mental Health Journal*, Vol. 19(2): 245–259.

Robert-Tissot, C., Cramer, B., Stern, D., Rusconi Serpa, S., Bachmann, J.P., Palacio Espasa, F., Knauer, D., De Muralt, M., Berney, C., and Mendigure, G. (1996). Outcome Evaluation in Brief Mother-Infant Psychotherapies: Report on 75 Cases. *Infant Mental Health Journal*, Vol. 17(2): 97–114.

Salomonsson, B. (2014). *Psychoanalytic Therapy with Infants and Parents*. London and New York: Routledge.

Stern- Bruschweiler, N., and Stern, D.N. (1989). A Model for Conceptualizing the Role of the Mother's Representational World in Various Mother-Infant Therapies. *Infant Mental Health Journal*, Vol. 10(3): 142–156.

Stern, D. (1995). *The Motherhood Constellation*. London: Karnac Books.

Stern, D. (1998). The Process of Therapeutic Change Involving Implicit Knowledge: Some Implications of Developmental Observations for Adult Psychotherapy. *Infant Mental Health Journal*, Vol. 19(3): 300–308.

Sternberg, J. (2005). *Infant Observation at the Heart of Training*. London: Karnac Books.

Thomson Salo, F. (2001). Some Principle of Infant-Parent Psychotherapy. *Australian Journal of Psychotherapy*, Vol. 20(1&2): 36–59.

Trad, P.V. (1993). *Short-Term Parent-Infant Psychotherapy*. New York: Basic Books.

Tzŭ, L. (2010, 500 BC). *Tao Tê Ching by Waley*. London: The Folio Society.

Tzŭ, L. (1999, 500 BC). *Tao Tê Ching (Book of the Way)*. (translated by Stephen Mitchell), p. 6. London: Frances Lincoln Ltd.

Watillon, A. (1993). The Dynamics of Psychoanalytic Therapies of the Early Parent-Child Relationship. *International Journal of Psycho-Analysis*, Vol. 74: 1037–1048.

Winnicott, D.W. (1941). The Observation of Infants in a Set Situation. *International Journal of Psychoanalysis*, Vol. 22: 229–249.

Woodhead, J., Bland, K., and Baradon, T. (2006). Focusing the Lens: The Use of Digital Video in the Practice and Evaluation of Parent-Infant Psychotherapy. *Infant Observation. The International Journal of Infant Observation and Its Applications*, Vol. 9(2): 139–150.

2   What is mindfulness?

This being human is a guest house.
Every morning a new arrival.
A joy, a depression, a meanness,
some momentary awareness comes
as an unexpected visitor.
Welcome and entertain them all!
Even if they're a crowd of sorrows,
who violently sweep your house
empty of its furniture,
still, treat each guest honorably.
He may be clearing you out
for some new delight.
The dark thought, the shame, the malice,
meet them at the door laughing,
and invite them in.
Be grateful for whoever comes,
because each has been sent
as a guide from beyond.
                         Rumi, circa 1250, p. 109

Simply speaking, mindfulness means "full of mind", where the word "mind", in Asian languages, does not refer merely to the intellect but also to the heart. Mindfulness can be equated to heartfulness (Kabat-Zinn, 1990, p. XXXV). It encompasses the complex meanings of awareness, observation, attention and remembering and describes a way of being. Mindfulness is translated from the Pali word *Sati*, the language used to record the Buddhist teaching. "[…] *sati*, is cultivated as a tool to observe how the mind [operates and often] creates suffering moment by moment. It is practiced to develop wisdom and insight, which ultimately alleviates suffering". (Siegel et al., 2010, p. 26). He continues:

Awareness is inherently powerful [...] and attention, which is focused awareness, is still more powerful. Just by becoming aware of what is occurring within and around us, we can begin to untangle ourselves from mental preoccupations and difficult emotions. [...] Another aspect of mindfulness is "remembering". This does not refer to memory of past events. Rather, it means remembering to be aware and pay attention, highlighting the importance of *intention* in mindfulness practice.

(Ibid., p. 18)

He invites us to remember to be aware and that: "[...] the purpose of mindfulness in its ancient context is to eliminate needless suffering by cultivating insight into the workings of the mind and the nature of the material world" (Ibid., p. 18).

Here below is my understanding of his view on mindfulness. It helps to calm the emotional and physical turmoil and allows us to clearly see our tangled emotions, which are in a constant, changing flow.

Awareness of impermanence is, indeed, one of the essential tenets of mindfulness and prevents us from being overwhelmed by fleeting states of mind.

Happiness is what we are all after, although we may have very different ideas of what happiness is and how to achieve it and – to some degree – to keep it. In her book on mindfulness Ruby Wax, comedienne and writer, trained in Mindfulness-Based Cognitive Therapy (MBCT), mentions old philosophers and thinkers, who were all concerned with defining happiness and moving towards obtaining it. She quotes from various sources including

> Seneca, "The only thing we own is our mind"; then Epicurus, "There are only three important ingredients to happiness: friendship, freedom (not to be owned by anyone), and an analysed life"; Aristoteles: "Happiness is the goal of goals"; then Nietzsche, "Great happiness requires great suffering"; Lincoln, "Most folks are as happy as they make up their mind to be"; the Buddha, 'Life is suffering [but he showed the way out of suffering]; and the XIV Dalai Lama, "Happiness is not something readymade. It comes from your actions."
>
> (Wax, 2016, p. 30)

Jon Kabat-Zinn, who has pioneered the application of mindfulness in hospitals, medical centres, clinics etc. in the USA, is well known for his short and sharp definition on mindfulness, which is "paying attention in a particular way: on purpose, in the present moment and nonjudgmentally" (Kabat-Zinn, 1994, p. 4). He writes, "Awareness requires only that we pay attention and see things as they are. It doesn't require that we change anything" (Kabat-Zinn, 1990, p. 20). The present moment is the only moment we have; past and future are just in the mind; only an open and receptive mind can see and learn in the present, then changes can happen. Purposeful implies that we know that we are practising mindfulness but we do not strive to achieve anything; we just are, just accept things as they are without criticising ourselves or others; without pursuing or expecting results; without feeling that we or things are right, wrong or neutral.

The whole being is brought to the process of mindfulness: the body, its sensory modalities, the physical sensations, the head with its habitual, repetitive churning of thoughts, the feeling heart with its endless string of positive, negative, neutral emotions are all involved in mindfulness practice. We befriend them and reconcile with them in an attitude of forgiveness, compassion and acceptance that all that is simply the way it is.

We talk of embodiment of mindfulness. Being still and noticing what goes on inside us as well as out there requires that we notice our breathing with its rising and lowering of the chest; our heartbeat and the loud or subtle sounds and noises around us. We see what goes on around us if our eyes are open; we smell odours and scents; we experience sensations of all sorts: from pain and stiffness to relaxation, to cold and warmth, tingling and numbness. We become aware of feeling alert, excited, elated, scared, tired, sleepy, bored, depressed, anxious, expectant and last but not least, our imagination kicks off and takes us into many realms and worlds filled with memories, dreams, plans, projects, thoughts and phantasies. At this point we lose the connection with the present moment, with our breathing and fly away from being in the body in the here and now: mindfulness is lost! But as we regain the awareness – with a benevolent and non-critical stance – of having moved out of both the present moment and the actual body, we are back to a mindful state, now fully conscious again of our mental wanderings. This is what mindfulness is about: a very old discipline and an ancient wisdom.

Psychiatrist Russell Razzaque in his slide presentation in a Child and Adolescent Mental Health Clinic (C.A.M.H.S.) in 2015, mentioned that in the 1980s a large amount of evidence around the so-called "third-wave therapies" – Mindfulness-based cognitiove therapy (MBCT), Dialectic Behaviour Therapy (DBT), Acceptance and Commitment Therapy (ACT) – started to emerge. They aimed at gaining awareness of the inner world of thoughts and emotions merely by observing them non-judgementally. By this simple act of observation, we are no longer reacting to experiences and by accepting them, we are no longer controlled by them. Mindfulness is a mainstream therapy recommended by National Institute of Clinical Excellence (NICE) and by numerous international advisory bodies. Razzaque confirmed that mindfulness is the rediscovery of ancient wisdom (Razzaque, 2015).

Mindfulness can be practised by all sorts of different people including small children, adolescents, parents, professionals etc. in all sort of settings, secular institutions and circumstances. There is now a vast movement called "Mindfulness in School", which has pioneered the teaching and practice of mindfulness with children in schools, adopting different techniques and strategies depending on their age. Teachers have a three-day-training programme to learn the mindfulness curriculum Paws B. (Pause and breath) for children aged seven to 11. Goodman and Greenland (2010, p. 418) write about programmes that bring mindfulness awareness practice to children in pre-kindergarten to secondary school pupils. This helps them to understand emotional turmoil, to calm down and regulate their feelings without reacting to, or being drowned by them, allowing them to let them go according to the principle of impermanence that everything passes and changes.

Psychiatrists, psychotherapists, psychologists and mental health practitioners have added mindfulness in their work with both children and adults as documented in the book by Pozzi Monzo: *The Buddha and the Baby* (2014).

Mindfulness has extended to the House of Parliament, where ministers Lawson and Ruane not only have embraced it personally but have managed to introduce it to their parliamentary colleagues. They explain their vision of how education policy might change to embrace the benefits of mindfulness. In Scotland, too, the chief medical officer Burns proposes the use of mindfulness in the social and health care sectors. In the United States congressman Ryan, who wrote a book called *A Mindful Nation*, also advocates the use of mindfulness in health care, education, the military and criminal justice (in Kabat-Zinn, ibid., pp. 237–8).

Mindfulness programmes called Vipassana training have been introduced in prisons in India, America and many other countries and have achieved unimaginable changes and "conversions" in callous criminals with life-long convictions for all sort of crimes, including murder (Vipassana DVD, Vipassana Research Institute, 1997). At the Tavistock Centre of Human Relationships in London mindfulness training is offered to staff working there and patients and is so described:

> Mindfulness is a very effective way of training our attention. In our fast-paced world, we are increasingly reacting automatically, too busy to notice much of what is going on inside or around us. By training our attention in a kindly way we can live more fully in the present, rather than brooding about the past or worrying about the future. Mindfulness helps reduce the power of unhelpful thoughts which are often "running the show". It helps us to connect more fully with our experiences and in time to better manage difficult thoughts and feelings.

Mindfulness is a popular, highly researched intervention with many applications that are demonstrated to have clear effects on the immune system and brain functioning. It can reduce physical and mental disorders such as stress and depression and it is also applied to treat addictions. In a further section, I will explore more the value and application of mindfulness in medical sciences.

Mindfulness techniques

A basic exercise to prepare the ground for further exercises, is mindful breathing. This can be done with children from the age of six, adolescents and adults. It helps to self-regulate i.e. to both down-regulate anxiety states by stimulating the parasympathetic nervous system or by up-regulating the hypo-arousal state and to achieve a felt state of calm and well-being.

In general, this starts with correct posture. Whether sitting on a cushion or on a chair, one's back has to be straight but equally relaxed with shoulders lowered and chin tucked into the neck. Hands are softly resting on one's lap or legs. It is best to keep one's eyes closed to avoid distraction from the surrounding environment. The attention is then placed on natural breathing, not controlled breathing; in particular it is focused at the base of the nose and the nostrils to facilitate feeling the physical sensation of the flow of air going in during inhalation, then going out during exhalation. One notices both the physical sensations in the whole body and the emotional feelings during these exercises. Distractions are inevitable as the nature of the mind is to jump from thought to thought, hence the need to rein it back firmly and un-judgementally to the focused point of attention, perhaps just by "noting" that one's thoughts are hopping around. This simple exercise of awareness requires ongoing practice and leads to a quieting of the churning mind and to a sense of peacefulness.

Another practice consists of body scanning where all the parts of one's body, including the internal organs, are focused upon, observed and named mentally, while breathing in and out. Again, this leads to a release of muscular tension and a general feeling of relaxation.

Mindful walking can be applied to both slow motion or ordinary walking and can be used in everyday life; also, mindfulness can be encouraged when standing waiting for the bus or train, or while doing ordinary household chores. Thus, increased awareness of the present moment becomes more habitual and reduces the growing hectic pace of our life.

Thich Nhat Hanh, the Buddhist monk leading the Buddhist Community of Plum Village in South France, wrote a book on mindfulness with children (2011). This described playful activities such as walking in the playground and stopping at the sound of a bell to visualise their breathing, then walking again when the bell sounds; tasting a raisin and being aware of the flavour, the sensation in the mouth, throat and stomach when swallowing the raisin; sitting in the lotus position and holding a little stone in their hand and with closed eyes feeling the sensations generated by the stone: hard, cold, warm, smooth, uneven etc. ...

Imaginative games can be proposed to the children such as thinking that they are the wind that blows on a meadow, or a flower standing and opening its petals; or watching a bus driving away on the road and comparing it to their emotions passing and not staying still.

These exercises can be very helpful for hyperactive children, for behavioural problems, anxieties and moods, eating disorders, phobias etc. They are also practised with the parents to begin with, so they can remind the children to practise them at home. Beneficial effects have occurred and outcomes have been validated by the widespread movement of Mindfulness in Schools.

Mindfulness and medical sciences

Many new and exciting discoveries have occurred in recent years in the area of medical sciences and the links between mind and body have no longer been seen to be so painfully separate as they were thought to be in the past. The neurosciences are showing us that the brain continues to grow and change all through life and in response to the external environment, as we will read throughout Chapter 2.

Kabat-Zinn (1990, p. 240) writes that there is an

> ever-increasing body of scientific evidence suggesting that MBSR [Mindfulness-Based Stress Reduction] and other mindfulness-based interventions can affect specific regions in the brain, positively influence at least certain immune functions, regulate emotions under stress, reduce pain, and improve a wide range of health indicators across many different medical diagnostic categories as well as in healthy individuals.

Amongst the fascinating discoveries in medical sciences that have occurred in the past few decades there are neuroplasticity, epigenesis and the discovery of telomeres.

(1) Neuroplasticity – the capacity to create new neural connections that are in continual communication – has demonstrated that the brain "is an organ of ongoing experience. It continues to grow and change and reshape itself across our entire life span in response to experience, right into old age" (Ibid., p. 219).

(2) The Greek word "epigenesis" literally means over and above (epi) the genome (that is the complete set of genes or genetic material present in a cell or organism) and it describes the mutual influence of genetic processes and environmental factors. Epigenetic is the study of biological mechanisms and heritable changes that will influence genetic processes by switching genes on and off; it is about the input of our experience, behaviour and lifestyle choices on our genetic endowment, which can be modified accordingly.

We are no longer imprisoned rigidly by our genetic heredity but can affect and modulate the expression of genes and influence our sensitivity to specific diseases. There is a well-known epigenetic study that suggests that when mother rats lick their pups, they leave epigenetic marks on their babies' DNA. This, in turn, helps them grow up to be calm adults. On the other hand, pups who receive very little licking, grooming, or nursing from their mothers tend to grow up more anxious. It was not their genes that dictated their stressed-out behaviour, but their epigenome, which was shaped by the nurturing behaviour of their mother. (https://en.wikipedia.org/wiki/Epigenetics)

(3) Kabat-Zinn writes about 2009 Nobel Prize winner Elizabeth Blackburn at the university of California, San Francisco, who discovered that

telomeres are structures [or enzymes that lengthen DNA segments, which ensure the stability of genetic material during cell division] at the end of all our chromosomes that are necessary for our cells to divide. The telomeres shorten a bit with each cell division, and over time, when they are completely gone, the cell can no longer replicate.

(Ibid., p. 220)

Stress shortens telomeres and so Blackburn and colleagues investigated the effect of mindfulness and other meditative practices on protecting against telomere shortening with good, early results.

It is now known that telomere length is directly related to ageing on the cellular level, and therefore, to how long we may live. The rate at which our telomeres degrade and shorten is very much affected by how much stress we are under and how well we cope with it.

(Ibid., p. 221)

We now know that the developing foetus and young babies' brains are very sensitive to stress and environmental factors that affect their healthy growth, their physiological and emotional development.

Mindfulness is "a core psychological process that can alter how we respond to the unavoidable difficulties in life – not only to everyday existential challenges, but also to severe psychological problems" (Siegal et al., 2010, p. 17).

Other authors have reported that, experiments within a healthy population demonstrated that experienced meditators – or in some cases even short-term meditators – compared with control groups of non-meditators, exposed to electroencephalograms (EEG) have shown a number of physical and psychological benefits. These range from decreased hypertension and blood pressure, reduced daily anxieties and changing moods to an increased capacity to moderate emotional arousal, better adaptation to stressful events, increase in antibody formation and improved immune system, better concentration and brain functioning. In an interesting study on the immune system, participants were given an influenza vaccine after the completion of mindfulness training and antibodies were measured at two time points, showing a greater increase in antibodies from time one to time two, compared with the control group (Kocovsky et al., 2010).

When practising mindfulness, anxieties, fears, panic, depression etc., are felt in the body, observed and acknowledged by naming them but without allowing them to take over one's life and preventing an ordinary adaptation to everyday events. These states are seen as flowing conditions of internal discomfort that will pass just like a train with its many carriages, that is being observed from a distance. This is one of the most common metaphors to describe mindfulness in simple terms.

Studies at the universities of Calgary, Bangor California have shown major improvements in patients with breast cancer and prostate cancer on physiological and psychological measures as a result of their cancer-oriented MBSR

(Mindfulness-based stress reduction) programme, writes Kabat-Zinn (2013, p. 257). The quality of life and its length has improved with decreased stress, blood pressure, mood disturbance, managing traumas etc., but also biological modifications have occurred such as modification in the immune system and in cortisol production. Didonna confirms that MBSR has shown efficacy not only in alleviating emotionally disturbed states, including sleep disturbance and other psychological stresses, but also in improving "biological regulation of a variety of circadian systems that are essential to promote health and homeostasis such as cytokine expression, cortical secretion, and blood pressure" (Carlson et al., 2010, p. 395).

Some severe eating disorders, Obsessive-Compulsive Disorders (OCD), suicidality, addictions, Post-Traumatic Stress Disorder (PTSD), borderline personalities, chronic pain management and even psychosis can all be ameliorated by training in any of the many forms of mindfulness-based interventions. Several authors in Didonna's *Clinical Handbook of Mindfulness*, have explored the application and – in some cases – the evidence-based results of mindfulness with various, severe disorders. Here follows a schematic but essential summary of these authors' ideas regarding these disorders and the effects of mindfulness practice. I will try to summarise the specific help offered by mindfulness to disorders beyond the increased, general attitude of feeling, observing, naming and letting go of emotions, sensations and thoughts.

Anxiety and fear are part of ordinary, everyday life and occur on a continuum that can provide stimulation to change and a boundary to danger; but when they become excessive and relentless, daily life is impaired. Greeson, J. and Brantley, J. (2010, p. 171) propose "a 'wise relationship' that develops by turning toward fear, anxiety, and panic with stable attention, present focused awareness, acceptance and self-compassion can promote psychological freedom from persistent anxiety and greater behavioral flexibility". Part of this "wise relationship" consists in re-perceiving one's anxieties and fears as transient conditions to be curious about without creating a story about them.

Obsessive-compulsive disorders (OCD) are chronic and often a severe psychiatric disease characterised – writes Didonna (Ibid., p. 189) – "by recurrent, intrusive and distressing thoughts, images, or impulses (obsessions) and/or repetitive mental or overt acts (compulsions or neutralizing behavior) performed to reduce or remove distress and anxiety". Because awareness of conscious thoughts during automatic, compulsive actions is lacking in people suffering with OCD, mindfulness may strengthen an anti-rumination process, improve the attentional deficit as well as increasing self-validation and acceptance to counterbalance the ongoing obsessive self-invalidation typical of these sufferers.

People who suffer from *major depression* and *suicidality* are oppressed by very negative thoughts about their past, present and future; have no interest in life and – being always tired – dread any possible pleasurable activity. The emphasis of MBCT is on helping participants to become aware and to disengage by responding differently to their negative, ruminative thoughts and feelings that may propel them even further into depression. These "third-wave therapies" are also particularly suitable for, and reduce risk of relapse in suicidal people by fostering the capacity to be open and see suicidal, intrusive thoughts as like any other thought or mental event – to be explored but not to be a source of fear or identification (Barnhofer and Crane, 2010).

Borderline personality disorder is a severe personality disorder presenting with difficulties in relationships, in regulating emotions and containing impulsive behaviours, in establishing a secure sense of identity not plagued by constant fear of abandonment, feelings of emptiness or dissociative moments with paranoid feelings. It is a condition that is difficult to treat, which often presents co-morbidity and puts huge strain on services and clinicians. Patients often drop out of treatment. However, Dialectic Behaviour Therapy (DBT) which has a strong component of mindfulness, has proved somewhat useful and it is based on acceptance of the patient and at the same time on pushing towards change with cognitive restructuring and skill training. This therapy has evidence-based results with this population. (Rizvi et al., 2010).

Eating disorders are characterised by deficit in self-regulation of food intake and difficulties in recognising signals of hunger; underlying this there is great difficulty in identifying emotions, in having a language to describe and manage them as well as distorted and rigid thinking about one's body image, weight, shape and appearance. Eating disorders are complex syndromes and persist even when physical and psychological deterioration continue. In view of their entrenched and multifaceted nature, innovative mindfulness-based therapies have been used together with traditional Cognitive Behavioural Therapy: Dialectical Behaviour Therapy (DBT). Acceptance and Commitment Therapy (ACT), MBCT and MB-EAT i.e. Mindfulness-Based Eating Awareness Training. This latter is based on guided imagery developed to address weight, shape and eating and self-regulatory issues. Its outcome indicates improvement in food intake, internalisation of the therapy and also biological changes in self-regulation (Wolevert and Best, 2010).

To seek pleasure and avoid pain is a normal tendency but the addict goes about it in a destructive and compulsive way with drugs, alcohol, gambling and sex. However, the pleasure thus provided is short-lived and compulsive patterns are established. *Addictive Behaviours* replace a pleasurable, pain-freeing activity with the discomfort of physiological withdrawal and the relentless need and dependence on something destructive and damaging to deal with further pain (Thomas Bien, 2010). Mindfulness can help to increase one's awareness of the destructive effects of the addiction and proposes changes to be taken with determination and appropriate actions towards a more satisfying lifestyle with an acceptance even of possible relapse urges seen as transitory and not fixed for ever and ever.

Mindfulness applied to *Post-Traumatic Stress Disorders and Traumas* proposes an alternative form of help to traditionally used exposure-based treatments, where memories and feelings of the traumatic event are re-activated and thought about. To help patients who may find the above approach impossible, mindfulness provides skills to help manage the distress felt during the exposure work. One skill consists in helping the person to let go of the need to control internal experiences, to increase self-regulation and cope-ability with negative feelings and to consider moving one's life in a more valued direction (Follette and Vijay, 2010).

ADHD is characterised by difficulty in attention, impulsivity, hyperactivity and seems to have an inherited, genetic component as well as psychological and environmental ones. It is a fast-spreading disorder in Europe and more so in the United States, affecting children from the age of seven and is being treated with both medications and psycho-social therapies. For those children and adults affected or at risk, mindful breathing as well as of walking have been proposed as additional tools to manage their hyperactivity. It helps them to feel more empowered by strengthening self-regulatory capacities and also alters the neurobiology of brain circuits in prefrontal cortex regions (Zylowska et al., 2010).

People suffering with *psychosis,* as well as presenting great suffering, have a poor insight into their illness, their mood instability, their bizarre ideations and behaviour and self- or outwardly directed violence. They are also resistant to traditional psychotherapies and pharmacological interventions are not always effective. The psychotic suffering is often increased by the patient's attitude towards the illness and the incomprehensibility of their delusional ideas and behaviour to them and the professionals. Mindfulness has to be explained to patients and the scope of it, which is not to prevent bad thoughts, voices, images from getting inside their mind, or disconcerting feelings of fragmentation and terror invading and taking them over. It aims at developing and observing with an attitude of curiosity, with no fear or judgement and to empower the patient to step back and not to act on their voices, thoughts and feelings. (Pinto, 2010, pp. 339–68).

Mindfulness is used for managing *chronic pain*, which can affect and impact on the physical and emotional well-being of a great number of adults.

> Chronic pain may be a warning that the body/mind has been challenged for too long or too intensely in some ways, and is not able to remain well, heal or cope beyond a certain level of physical or emotional stress, which may be cumulative.
>
> (Gardner-Fix, 2010, p. 378)

Training in mindfulness requires both the acceptance of the pain and its ensuing disability and the struggle to re-establish the earlier pain-free state.

Fulton writes about the "contribution mindfulness practice makes to the *mind of therapist*, and through it, to the therapy" itself. It helps the therapist "to cultivate mental capacities and qualities such as attention, affect tolerance, acceptance, empathy, equanimity, tolerance of uncertainty, insight into narcissistic tendencies, and perspective on the possibility of happiness" (Fulton, 2010, p. 408).

Mindfulness in my work with parents and infants

As a parent-infant psychotherapist working in public services, I have added a useful and complementary tool to help parents with babies referred for all

sorts of difficulties. First-time parents and also seasoned parents are often con-
fronted with anxious, unknown and bewildering situations, either when their baby
is growing in the womb or when the babies are out in the world. As well as offering the traditional psychoanalytically informed parent-infant psychotherapy – as
described in the previous chapter – I propose mindfulness also described in the
above section: *Mindfulness techniques*. An important aim in using this technique
is to allow them to see the baby as a separate being, as a little person with his or
her own mind

I was once asked by an uninitiated colleague of mine, when in my therapy
I would introduce mindfulness. That was an interesting question which I had
never considered, as I had introduced this method spontaneously up to that
time. The moment when mindfulness is introduced often follows an intuitive
response to something in the session.

However, in paying more attention to when I offer mindfulness techniques,
some circumstances came to mind. For example, if mothers or fathers "tell" me
something about family life, baby's problems, marital issues but in a detached
and unemotional way, I may then introduce mindfulness to invite the parent to
focus on the bodily sensations as well as on the emotions and feelings going
through them.

This was the case with a very insightful mother, who already had understood
intellectually a lot about her own and her baby's predicament and yet the feelings were not there, and the original difficulty could not be resolved. We understood the need to defend herself from painful feelings regarding her painful
story and gradually feelings began to flow and the symptoms went away. An
almost opposite situation is when the story is poured out by the parent in an
uncontained flow and evacuated with no pause. Then, mindfulness can be very
useful to stop this running on and allow pauses, just like when hyperactive children are invited to pause and breathe (see above: on mindfulness exercises with
children). Again, the psychic pain avoided by this running on can be looked at
within the psychotherapeutic work.

Some parents are lacking in insight, through no fault of their own, and want
something practical to help them. Mindfulness in relation to themselves and
also applied to observing their infant, can open up ways to understanding their
baby and to learning about their mutual interactions.

In a situation of impasse in a session, when neither the parent nor myself, the
therapist, have much to say but are respectively paralysed with fears and anxieties or intense projections from the parent, mindfulness can rescue both of us. It
can prove an effective tool to unblock the impasse and allow the flow of communication to resume.

A last value of this technique that I am aware of, is that of giving parents
a concrete, practical tool to take away, together with the more impalpable ideas
that emerge in sessions. They can practice mindfulness in their own time and
with their babies, perhaps at fraught and tired moments in their daily life.

Still as part of my work, I have gathered a few groups of mothers and
babies (fathers are rarely available due to work commitments) either in the

clinic or in the children's centre and offered them to be part of a mindfulness group for mothers and babies. In these group sessions we all sit comfortably on a cushion on a floor mat provided. Mothers are asked to place their baby in their lap or cradled between their crossed legs facing them. The first 10–15 minutes are spent practising mindful breathing and scanning the body to encourage them to get in touch with different parts of their bodies, to really notice if they are holding any tension and then to actively direct the breath into those areas of tension. They are asked to become aware of any physical sensations starting from the head, the forehead, the face etc., down to the toes. They have to focus on their breathing without forcing it and to notice how their breath has become deeper and slower. They are asked to observe their baby lying in their lap, just to observe them, not to play, nor jiggle them nor coo to them. It is not easy to begin with and just to be and to observe oneself and one's baby, to do nothing, and to maintain sharp awareness without falling asleep.

Amongst the benefits of these groups for either parents who are referred for any problem to the clinic or for those parents who are regularly going to children centres and are just curious to try mindfulness, are an increased sense of well-being and relaxation, that is fed back by parents after the mindfulness practice. They also notice how their fretful baby may have calmed down or fallen asleep after hours of whining and whingeing or started feeding after turning away from the bottle or in one case, being able to "miraculously poo", while mother was breathing rhythmically and massaging the baby's badly constipated tummy.

In the next chapter, I will explore how the brain is formed – starting from uterine life – how it works and how mindfulness can bring changes to its functioning.

Bibliography

Barnhofer, T., and Crane, C. (2010). Mindfulness-Based Cognitive Therapy for Depression and Suicidality. In Didonna (2010a), pp. 221–243.

Bien, T. (2010). Paradise Lost: *Mindfulness and Addictive Behavior.* In Didonna (2010a), pp. 289–297.

Carlson, L.E., Labelle, L.E., Garland, S.L., Hutchins, M.L., and Birnie, K. (2010). *Mindfulness-Based Interventions in Oncology*, pp. 383–404.

Didonna, F. (2010a). *Clinical Handbook of Mindfulness.* New York: Springer Publisher.

Didonna, F. (2010b). *Mindfulness and Obsessive-Compulsive Disorders: Developing a Way to Trust and Validate One's Internal Experience*, pp. 189–219.

Follette, V.M., and Vijay, A. (2010). Mindfulness and Borderline Personality Disorder. In Didonna (2010a), pp. 299–317.

Fulton, P.R. (2010). Mindfulness-Based Intervention in an Individual Clinical Setting: What Difference Mindfulness Makes behind Closed Doors. In Didonna (2010a), pp. 407–416.

Gardner-Fix, J. (2010). Mindfulness-Based Stress Reduction for Chronic Pain Management. In Didonna (2010a), pp. 369–581.

Goodman, T.A., and Greenland, S.K. (2010). Mindfulness with Children: Working with Difficult Emotions. In Didonna (2010a), pp. 417–429.

Greeson, J., and Brantley, J. (2010). Mindfulness and Anxiety Disorders: Developing a Wise Relationship with the Inner Experience of Fear. In Didonna (2010a), pp. 171–188.

Kabat-Zinn, J. (1990). *Full Catastrophe Living*. UK: Piatkus Publisher.

Kabat-Zinn, J. (1994). *Wherever You Go, There You Are: Mindfulness Meditation in Everyday Life*. New York: Hyperion.

Kocovsky, N.L., Segal, Z.V., and Battista, S.R. (2010). Mindfulness and Psychopathology: Problem Formulation. In Didonna (2010a), pp. 90–91.

Pozzi Monzo, M. (2014). *The Buddha and the Baby*. London: Karnac Books.

Pinto, P. (2010). Mindfulness and Psychosis. In Didonna (2010a), pp. 339–368.

Razzaque, R. (2015). Slide Presentation.

Rizvi, S.L., Shaw, W.S., and Dimidjian, S. (2010). Mindfulness and Borderline Personality Disorder. In Didonna (2010a), pp. 245–257.

Rumi. (circa 1250) (1995). The Guest House. In: *The Essential Rumi*, p. 109. Translated by Coleman Barks with John Moyne. London: Penguin Books.

Siegal, R.D., Germer, C.K., and Olendzki, A. (2010). Mindfulness: What Is It? Where Did It Come From? In Didonna (2010a), pp. 17–35.

Thich Nhat Hanh. (2011). *Planting Seeds. Practicing Mindfulness with Children*. Berkley, CA: Parallax Press.

Vipassana Research Institute. (1997). *Doing Time, Doing Vipassana*. www.prison.dhamma.org. DVD available at email address: bookstore@pariyatti.org.

Wolevert, R.Q., and Best, J.L. (2010). Mindfulness-Based Approaches to Eating Disorders. In Didonna (2010a), pp. 259–287.

Wax, R. (2016). *A Mindfulness Guide for the Frazzled*. UK: Penguin Life.

Zylowska, L., Smalley, S.L., and Schwartz, J.M. (2010). Mindfulness Awareness and ADHD. In Didonna (2010a), pp. 319–338.

3   The development of the infant's brain and nervous system

As human beings we are basically all the same;
after all we all belong to the same planet.
All sentient beings have the same innate nature
that wants happiness and doesn't want to suffer.
All of us love ourselves and desire something good.

The Dalai Lama, 2000

In recent decades, the brain has become an object of great interest and study in the scientific world and, in particular, how the physical brain and the mind affect each other and impact on our health. The plasticity of the brain allows it to grow and change not just with every encounter, experience and thought but also into old age; new neurons as well as synaptic connections can be generated in response to our daily experiences or pruned if not used.

The times of maximal brain growth and change are in the last trimester of pregnancy and into the first two-to-three years of life

Neurons, trillions of them, send electrical signals to each other triggering the release of neurotransmitters and the production of hormones such as adrenaline, noradrenaline and cortisol by the adrenal and pituitary glands. They transmit information and trigger responses in cells and tissues. If behaviours, thoughts and feelings are repeated over and over, the neural connections become hard-wired and habits are created. This echoes Bion's clinical notions of container and contained, where the repetition of containing experiences by the parental primary carer becomes internalised by the infant, who learns to self-regulate and contain himself.

The brain can be divided into three parts, or we can say that there are three brains: the oldest one, the reptilian brain, which is in charge of our basic bodily functions such as breathing, heart beating, digestive processes, raw emotions etc.; around the reptilian brain, the limbic brain has developed. Its function consists in registering, analysing and remembering the strong emotions and drives coming from the reptilian brain. The third brain called neo-mammalian brain or neo-cortex, is located around the two brain hemispheres and is in charge of self-regulation, impulse control, insight, problem-solving, attention, empathy and thinking about thinking. These three brain parts are necessary and linked with each another.

The autonomic nervous system regulates the internal states of the body such as the heart rate, blood pressure and the digestive processes. It is divided in two branches or systems: the sympathetic nervous system and the parasympathetic one. The sympathetic system stimulates and is activated in both the fight-or-flight and freeze reaction; it tends to speed up activities, for example, it stimulates the heartbeat, the muscular tension, the dilating of the pupil and heightening of sense perceptions, etc. when we react to stress.

The fight-or-flight reaction is very helpful in threatening situations and has been of fundamental importance in our evolutionary survival. However, as we will see in Chapter 3, when we cannot modulate it or use it when there is no immediate threat to life or well-being, our fight-or-flight pathways

> can become chronically activated [...] and they change our biology as well as our psychology. We become primed, so to speak, for all the problems associated with hyperarousal right down to the level of which genes in our chromosomes get turned on and upregulated, such as the gene for the glucocorticoid receptors that make us chronically susceptible to stressors, and the genes that produce pro-inflammatory cytokines, which themselves promote a whole range of diseases of inflammation if chronically stimu-lated. Chronic arousal also shortens our telomeres, [...] and thus accelerates the ageing process at cellular level.
>
> (Kabat-Zinn, 1990, p. 318)

In the limbic area there is a small, almond-shaped cluster of neurons called the amygdala. Wax describes the amygdala as "the emergency button for our fight-flight or freeze response" (2016, p. 62) when there is a danger. It triggers a series of chemical messengers to activate our endocrine system; namely, the hormones adrenaline and cortisol useful to our organism but toxic if in exces-sive quantity. Adrenaline increases the heartbeat and blood pressure, while corti-sol suppresses the immune system and weakens the neurons connection with each other in some areas of the brain (hippocampus). "If the sympathetic state persists, the neurons wither and die, especially those in the area of memory" (Ibid., p 64), hence the mind goes blank and one cannot remember much.

> Every thought produces biochemical reactions in the brain, which match a feeling in the body. When you think happy thoughts, the body feels good, thanks to the power of dopamine; you think sad, you feel sad. The brain picks up bodily emotions and translates them into thoughts.
>
> (Ibid., p. 64)

A cycle is established: feelings to thinking, thinking to feelings. When we think differently, our brain can also be different and change.

A counter-regulatory switch occurs when the parasympathetic nervous system is turned on and dampens the hyperarousal of the sympathetic system. It slows down and calms activities such as body temperature, heartbeat, blood pressure and acts as a brake and a calm state is re-established in the body. The vagus nerve (the Latin origin of the name means wandering) is part of the parasympathetic nervous system and plays an important role in how we manage stress: the higher the level of stress the lower the activation of the vagal nerve. Kabat-Zinn writes

> Having a higher vagal tone is associated with greater calm and resilience, as well as recovering from stress more rapidly, greater social engagement, and positive emotions. Interestingly enough, just bringing awareness to your breathing and allowing it to slow down on its own, particularly the outbreaths, increases vagal tone.
>
> (Ibid., p. 314)

Infants, children and adults with good vagal tone manage ordinary and stressful situations calmly, can self-regulate, are happier and generally well settled in their life.

We can train our attention to focus on bodily sensations and feelings moment by moment, thus reducing the endless churning of the mind and containing the tendency to have full-blown reactions. We can choose, to a certain extent, which nervous system to switch on and how to move from a sympathetic-type reaction to a parasympathetic-type response. We can learn to respond mindfully rather than react mindlessly even in stressful situations.

Below is a brief description of brain areas, its schematic structure and how the functioning of different brain areas is affected by mindfulness practice (Figure 3.1).

> [The] Grey Matter holds most of the brain cells, and if it increases in density, it means that there's an increase in connectivity between the neurons [...] and their density determines the vitality and strength of your thinking. Mindfulness promotes the growth of grey matter in many regions of the brain.
>
> (Wax, Ibid., p. 68)

The Prefrontal Cortex (PFC) is the cerebral cortex that covers the front part of the frontal lobe. This region of the brain performs the so-called executive functions such as planning complex cognitive behaviours, making decisions, differentiating between conflicting thoughts, managing emotional control, social attachment and antisocial impulses, using empathy and, in general, self-regulating. Mindfulness increases this area of the brain.

The Amygdala, located in the temporal lobe of the limbic system, is central to fear responses and is activated when there is a sense of threat or danger; it has a function in processing memory, decision-making and emotional responses. It becomes less active with mindfulness practice (Luts et al. in Music, 2015).

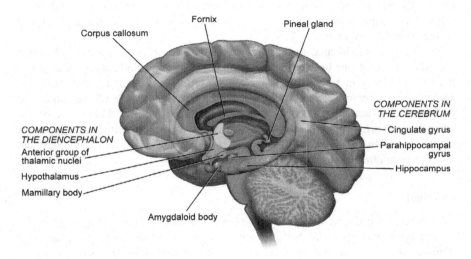

Corpus callosum
Fornix
Pineal gland

COMPONENTS IN THE CEREBRUM
Cingulate gyrus
Parahippocampal gyrus
Hippocampus

COMPONENTS IN THE DIENCEPHALON
Anterior group of thalamic nuclei
Hypothalamus
Mamillary body

Amygdaloid body

Figure 3.1 The Limbic System. Courtesy of Blausen.com staff (2014). "Medical gallery of Blausen Medical 2014". WikiJournal of Medicine 1 (2). DOI:10.15347/wjm/ 2014.010. [ISSN 2002–4436]

The Insula, located in the lateral sulcus of the cerebral cortex, fosters the awareness and processing of our bodily sensations and emotions, creating an ability to stand back and watch thoughts and feelings; it apparently grows bigger with the practice of mindfulness.

The Hippocampus, located under the cerebral cortex in the limbic system, plays an important role in consolidating information from short-term memory to long-term memory, in spatial memory and navigation. Mindfulness increases concentration of grey matter and structural changes thus improving "mental dexterity, flexibility of thinking and memory recall." (Wax, 2016, p. 69).

The Anterior Cingulate Cortex (ACC), located around the corpus callosus and connected to the prefrontal cortex, plays a function in regulating heart rate and blood pressure and is also involved in higher-level functions such as self-regulation, decision-making, holding focus in the face of distractions, controlling distress and switching "focus from the thinking mind to the feeling mind" (Ibid.). It is a conduit between the cognitive functions of the prefrontal cortex and the emotional experiences of the limbic system; it shows increased activation when sadness is induced (https://en.wikipedia.org/wiki/Anterior_cingulate_ cortex). Mindfulness has proved to strengthen attention regulation.

The Temporo-Parietal Junction, located between the temporal and the parietal lobes, integrates information from the external environment as well as from within the body and brain and processes them. It provides the ability to orient the body in space and to feel located within one's body. It plays a role in emotional processing, ethical and moral decision-making and has a crucial role in the theory of mind, which has now been proved to have a neural basis (https://en.wikipedia.org/wiki/Temporoparietal_junction). Brain imaging shows an increase in grey matter in this area.

Mirror Neurons, located in the Broca's area of the frontal lobe in the Inferior Parietal Cortex of our brain, were first identified by Rizzolatti and colleagues at Parma University in Italy. This is thought to represent one of the most important findings of neurosciences in the last decades. Every time we see someone performing an action, the same neurons and motor circuits that are activated when we perform that same action, are activated at the same time as the person we observe. This makes us able to reflect and synchronise with the feelings we observe in another person standing in front of us.

Cortisol

Now a few words on cortisol, the steroid hormone often nicknamed as the "stress hormone". Cortisol has the potential to inhibit areas of the brain that regulate attention and can weaken the activity of the immune system and also bone density. It is released in response to stress and low blood-glucose concentration. It increases the risk of depression and mental illnesses. It is apparently

> a major threat to the healthy development of a child's brain. Produced by the adrenal glands, cortisol helps the human body respond in a time of crisis by moderating its level of stress-response, but elevated levels of this hormone interfere with the building of neural pathways and may even have the effect of dissolving established connections.
>
> (Ladnier and Massnari, 2000, p. 37)

Talge and colleagues write that "lower concentrations of cortisol secretion have been associated with PTSD, whereas higher concentrations have been associated with generalised anxiety disorder as well as depression" (Talge et al., 2007, p. 253). There is a correlation between stress in mothers during pregnancy and post-natal development of the infant. Elevation in maternal cortisol concentrations "have been associated with both lower birth weights and elevated glucocorticoid levels in offspring" (Ibid., p. 246). Babies born to mothers with high levels of anxiety show greater right-frontal brain activity, which is associated with negative affect from infancy and all through one's life span. These babies spend more time in deep sleep and less in an active and alert state and perform poorly on the Neonatal Behavioral Assessment Scale (NBAS) and on the Bayley Mental Developmental Index (MDI), Talge et al. write (Ibid., p. 253). "The hypothalamic-pituitary-adrenal (HPA) axis in both mother and child [is] the primary biological mechanism underlying long-term effect of prenatal stress" (Ibid., p. 253). Also, the authors continue, early post-natal experiences affect the developing cortico-limbic circuits involved in the regulation of the HPA, increasing the vulnerability to stress. Babies who have been subjected to maternal stress during pregnancy tend to be particularly anxious, to freeze and lack in exploratory behaviour, spatial memory and some aspects of cognitive functioning, which are typical of a high concentration of cortisol. However, post-natal environment, the authors continue with a hopeful note, can reverse the effects of perinatal stress at a behavioural and cognitive level.

Music (2014) writes that when people are emotionally overwhelmed, anxious and frightened, the subcortical limbic system with the amygdala, is activated and prevents access to the prefrontal self-reflective brain and its executive functions of self-reflectiveness and self-awareness. Emanuel (2004) also reflects on the neurobiological effect of childhood trauma, when the fear pathway and the fight-or-flight response are activated in sub-thalamic behaviour with an over-production of cortisol and the inhibition of the prefrontal cortex. In a personal communication, he also refers to the new discoveries that the brain does not have a dedicated region or network for psychological phenomena such as thinking, feeling, deciding and seeing as Lisa Feldman Barret revealed. The question is now how is an emotion created by the brain?

Parents who are anxious, tense, have been abused, traumatised and been the object of domestic violence, transmit in a totally unconscious and neurologically fixed fashion, similar emotional states to their babies. These in turn, respond by being fretful, restless, whingeing, whimpering etc. This is a familiar scenario with mothers and fathers referred with their babies to perinatal and parent-infant services. Parent-infant psychotherapy and mindfulness offer containment and understanding by increasing self-reflective awareness and performing also a neurophysiological rebalancing of the amygdala and linking of the subcortical emotion brain with the cortical, executive brain.

The developing brain of the infant

I am grateful to Balbernie (2001), Pally (2000) and Schore (2001) for their very clear and comprehensive writing on how early relationship experiences affect the forming and developing brain of the infant during pregnancy and in the first two-to-three years of the young child's life. This is the optimal period for synaptic production and rapid brain growth and development. The cerebral cortex, begins to form from the 24th week of gestation and into the first year of life becoming thicker and richer in neuronal connections. Pally writes, "For the nine months of gestation and for a few months after birth, brain growth and development is largely directed by the genetic code" (2000, p. 4) *"In utero* development provides only an approximate sketch of the wiring of the topographically arranged visual cortex. The more precise wiring requires stimulation from post-natal sensory experiences." (Pally, 1997, p. 590). She writes that the myelin sheet that allows fast conduction of impulses in the cell axon begins soon after birth and in the first months of life; the prefrontal cortex begins to myelinate at about three months and into young adulthood. Balbernie writes: "The postnatal period is marked by a huge sequential proliferation and over-production of a number of synapses; this is under the control of genes activated by experience" (Balbernie, 2001, p. 240). In this period about two million new synapses are generated in a second.

A functioning synapse is formed when the axon of one neuron hooks onto the dendrite of another. [...] This is done by neurotransmitters, chemicals that enable the synapse to conduct electrical impulses between the neurons. [...] In the first few years of life each neuron forms about 15.000 synapses. By the age of two the child has as many synapses as an adult, and by age three this has doubled to about 1.000 trillion.

(Ibid.)

The baby's brain at birth is designed to change in response to external signals, and as the brain develops,

it can respond to new experiences and thus develop further. [...] The prime task of brain development in the first few years of life is the forming, and then reinforcing into permanence, of necessary connections. The baby must interact with a living and responsive environment in order to ensure normal brain growth.

(Ibid., p. 239)

The stabilised synapses will survive while those which were not used enough will disappear. The

production and pruning of synapses is a use dependent fashion in the first few years of life [and] enables children to fit in to whatever circumstances surround them; examples of this process are the rapid patterning of relationships and self-control, as well as the speed at which the phonetics and grammar of language are acquired.

(Ibid., p. 241)

It is the quality and the quantity of emotional relationship with the primary figure that determines the forming and the losing of neural connections.

In the first year of life, the orbitofrontal cortex, which is very much affected by the quality of parental care, becomes active for affect regulation and communication through eye contact becomes very important. Already aged two months, the infant shows a vivid interest in the mother's face, eyes and pupils which "acts as a nonverbal communication device" (Hesse in Schore, 2001, p. 303) stimulating the infant's cognitive and social attunement to the mother. At around nine months, with a maturation of the limbic and cortical areas, the infant begins to have a theory of mind and becomes aware of the other person's states of mind. Neural networks in the orbitofrontal cortex are "sensitive to body language, face-to-face communication, tone of voice and eye contact". (Balbernie, 2001, p. 244). Talking to one's infant, showing lively facial expressions, playing animatedly and relating to the infant as someone who can understand and respond to the emotional communication, become an important and essential aspect of building a healthy mind-body relationship with the baby. During these exchanges, the maternal figure will co-modulate the infant's excitement.

In the second year of life, another "cortico-limbic circuit is established in the right hemisphere to regulate negative feelings. This second circuit is influenced by parental disapproval" (Balbernie, Ibid., p. 244). The 18-month-old toddler begins to have a sense of himself, to use personal pronouns, to recognise him/herself in the mirror and to develop an autobiographical memory.

Different brain areas process different input from the environment i.e. colours, sounds, motions, contour and the memory of these features, writes Pally. These areas "are richly connected to other brain regions by interconnecting neurons that form re-entry circuits" (Pally, 2000, p. 7). Through this re-entry process,

> the brain co-ordinates the information from these separate stimulus processing regions. For example, information processed in the visual cortex automatically influences processes in the auditory cortex and vice versa. Thus, what you see will influence what you hear and what you hear will influence what you see.
>
> (Ibid., p. 8)

This is very important as children who suffer from autism are often unable to pay attention to more than one sensory modality or one activity at a time: either they look or hear or pay attention or speak (Pozzi, 1993).

Another interesting aspect which has clinical relevance is the brain's different speed responses to environmental input, described by Pally (2000). In the quick, short response, the sensory stimuli go from the sense organ, for example the retina, through the thalamus and directly to the amygdala, which initiates survival behaviours. This bypasses the cortex and consciousness is not involved. The long and slower route travelled by the stimuli, goes from the thalamus to the sensory cortex, to the hippocampus and to the amygdala and orbitofrontal cortex. This "longer slower system involves the cortex and therefore can include conscious awareness." (Pally, p. 36). Psychotherapy and mindfulness provide an opportunity to transform the initial, reactive physical-emotional reaction into a more thoughtful physical-emotional response, using the longer route in the brain, allowing thinking to take place and considering the actual situation more correctly.

And on a lighter side, Ruby Wax (2016) writes;

> It is never too late to rethink your thinking. This means even if your parents screwed you up, nurturing experiences later in life can dramatically revise your biological make up, triggering different genes to switch on or off. It's not too late to change yours and your baby's gene expression.
>
> (p. 116)

Children "will inherit specific genes but everything that happens to them, starting with your interactions, will strike or silence those genes, determining their future abilities and traits" (Ibid.).

To summarise, repeated exposure to stimulation can either lead to habituation, where the same level of stimulation reduces the response, or to sensitisation, where the response is increased, genes are activated and new synapses are formed. The brain grows with appropriate environmental influences and the environment affects the expression of genes. (Pally, 1997 p. 591). Apparently, babies who receive more cuddles show genetic changes in their brain.

"Since it is known that consciously attending to and verbalising something can enhance cortical activation, it could theoretically be argued that treatments such as analysis enhance cortical functioning, and take advantage of cortical plasticity, to modulate deeply engrained emotional responses" (Pally, 2000, p. 15).

Emotions and feelings

Emotions, writes Damasio, "are complicated collections of chemical and neural responses, forming a pattern; all emotions have some regulatory role to play, [...] are about the life of an organism, its body to be precise, and their role is to assist the organism in maintaining life; [...] emotions are biologically determined processes depending on innately set brain devices, laid down by a long evolutionary history" (Damasio, 2000, p. 51). He continues,

> The devices which produce emotions occupy a fairly restricted ensemble of subcortical regions, beginning at the level of the brain stem, moving up to the hypothalamus, basal forebrain and amygdala; the devices are part of a set of structures that both regulate and represent body states.
>
> (Ibid.)

and these "devices can be engaged automatically, without conscious deliberation" (Ibid.). Most of our emotional responses are the result of an evolutionary process and "are part of the bioregulatory devices with which we come equipped to survive" (Ibid., p. 53). Darwin catalogued the emotional expressions of many species in many parts of the world and found consistency, and this allowed emotions to be recognised cross-culturally. Damasio separates

> three stages of processing along a continuum: *a state of emotion,* that can be triggered and executed nonconsciously; *a state of feeling,* which can be represented nonconsciously; and *a state of feelings made conscious,* i.e., known to the organism having both emotion and feeling.
>
> (p. 37)

Damasio describes the biological functions of emotions: one being the production of the flight-or-fight reaction in danger situations and the second one being the regulation of the internal state of our organism, such as to provide increased blood flow in case of having to run or change the heart and breathing rate in case of freezing. Emotions are part of our homeostatic regulation and become feelings when they are represented mentally and become conscious: we know that we have a feeling of an emotion. "Feelings are inwardly directed and private [...] mental expression of an emotion" (Damasio, Ibid., p. 36 and 42) and one can observe emotions but not feelings in someone else. "Consciousness allows feelings to be known and thus promotes the impact of emotions internally, allows emotions to permeate the thought process through the agency of feeling" (Ibid., p. 56). This is very important in the mindfulness process and in work with parents and babies, as we will read in the following chapters.

Here below, I am referring to further detailed studies, research and evidence about the long-term effects of mindfulness on brain function and structure. Again, I am grateful to both Ruby Wax (2016) for her clear, explanatory writing, and Fabrizio Didonna (2010) for his scientific exploration on this topic.

Effects of mindfulness on the brain

An increasing number of

> MRI studies of the impact of mindfulness suggest that it reliably and profoundly alters the structure and function of the brain to improve the quality of both thoughts and feelings. Mindfulness meditation appears to reshape the neural pathways, increasing the density and complexity of connections in areas associated with both cognitive abilities, such as attention, self-awareness and introspection, and emotional areas connected with kindness, compassion and rationality, while decreasing activity and growth in those areas involved with anxiety, hostility, worry and impulsivity.
>
> (Davidson quoted in Wax, 2016, pp. 83–4)

Research on meditators versus non-meditators published by the US National Institute of Health showed a 23% decrease in mortality over a 19-year period and 30% decrease in cardiovascular mortality in meditators. (Davidson, ibid.).

EEG recordings measure changes in electrical activity within the brain during mindfulness practice and can distinguish between different electrical frequencies produced by different brain activities. Short-term and long-term changes in neural functioning are likely to occur, according to studies (Treadway et al., 2010, p. 50), and such changes can take place in the individual while actively meditating and also over time as a result of regular practice. An individual's attentional capacity increases and the habituation – which is the tendency to reduce neural activity when the stimulus has been repeated many times – decreases. This means that attention can be sustained despite the presence of distracting stimuli. The findings show that different types of mindfulness practices produce different results but they support the evidence that meditation can promote changes in neural functioning.

> Meditation practices that emphasise deep physical relaxation are more likely to produce higher theta and delta activity (which are more closely associated

with deep sleep), while practices that focus more on intensive concentration and mindfulness will likely have higher alpha and beta power.

(Treadway and Lazar, 2010 p. 49)

Neuroimaging studies have achieved consistent findings. One is the activation of the dorsolateral prefrontal cortex (DLPFC), an area associated with executive decision-making and attention. Another finding is about the activation of the anterior subdivision of the cingulate cortex (ACC), which plays a role in the integration of attention, resolution of conflicts, emotional self-control and adaptive responses to changes, motivation and motor control (Didonna, 2010). The insula, which is associated with interoception i.e. visceral and gut feelings and contributes to our experience of selfness, is activated during mindfulness. Findings suggest that "abnormalities in insular function may play a critical role in various psychiatric disorders". (Treadway and Lazar, 2010, p. 51) In general, experiments with high resolution MRI images show increased cortical thickness in the anterior insula, sensory cortex and prefrontal cortex in the brain of long-term meditators. "Given the emphasis on observing internal sensations that occurs during meditation, thickening in this region is consistent with reports of mindfulness practice" (Ibid.).

A different form of mindfulness, which is based on naming of the affect experienced i.e. anger, sadness etc., and requires cognitive work, correlates with enhanced prefrontal regulation of affect.

But what are the neural mechanisms lying beyond the effects produced by mindfulness? Tentative fMRI research is investigating the neural impact of self-awareness focused on two forms of self-referential experiences: one is the momentary self-awareness, which is focused on the present experience; the second is the extended self-reference related to enduring characteristics and traits of the person. The "data suggest that one possible mechanism of action for mindfulness meditation is the decoupling of two self-referential neural networks that are normally integrated, and the strengthening of the experiential network" (Ibid., p. 52). If mindfulness can help people decouple their present moment experience from their long-term narrative sense of themselves ("I am fat, tall" etc.) even at a neural level, this may explain how this helps focussing on the current experience rather than on thoughts related with the past or future.

Wax reports "computer-based testing to measure the attentional performance of a group of medical and nursing students at the University of Pennsylvania, Philadelphia, before and after an eight-week mindfulness-based training course" (Wax, 2016, p. 54). Those who were taught mindfulness could direct and focus their attention more quickly; another study showed an increase in the ability to resist distraction. Further, Wax reports that Harvard neuroscientist Sara Lazar using fMRI found that the amount of grey matter in the insula increased in those who practiced mindfulness (Ibid., p. 71).

It is reported that Davidson and colleagues compared EEG patterns in healthy subjects before and after an eight-week training in mindfulness with a control group; they found differences in the EEG patterns; most important changes were correlated with improved immune function (Treadway and Lazar, 2010, p. 53).

We read that experienced meditators have higher frontal alpha asymmetry, which is associated with affective responding and particular patterns of asymmetry can be found in depression. Also, they have greater encephalogram coherence, which is indicative of brain coherence, intelligence, creativity and mental health (Kocovsky, et al., 2010, pp. 89–90). Further EEG studies found better capacity to moderate emotional arousal with long-term meditation; increased sensory acuity, decreased systolic blood pressure and brain response to pain in long-term meditators; while short-term meditation experience can bring about improved brain functioning. Improved immune system function, decrease in rumination, more balanced affective response and no relapse into depression were found in the sample of meditators and was due to a more balanced prefrontal activation.

Mindfulness requires one to focus and pay attention in the present moment non-judgementally and thus contains the wandering, anxious mind. It also emphasises acceptance and tolerance of the status quo and of possible symptoms, rather than suppressing or avoiding the present experience; this fosters emotional and psychological well-being.

Many more studies that demonstrate the effect of mindfulness are now proliferating, showing reduced reactivity to negative experiences, increased vitality and prolonged longevity even at a cellular level.

Bibliography

Balbernie, R. (2001). Circuits and Circumstances: The Neurobiological Consequences of Early Relationship Experiences and How They Shape Later Development. *Journal of Child Psychotherapy*, Vol. 27(10): 237–255.

Damasio, A. (2000). *The Feeling of What Happens*. London: Heinemann.

Didonna, F. (2010). *Clinical Handbook of Mindfulness*. New York: Springer Publisher.

Emanuel, R. (2004). Thalamic Fear. *Journal of Child Psychotherapy*, Vol. 30(1): 71–87.

Kabat-Zinn, J. (1990). *Full Catastrophe Living*. UK: Piatkus Publisher.

Kocovski, N.L., Segal, Z.V., and Battista, S.R. (2010). Mindfulness and Psychopathology: Problems Formulation. In: *Clinical Handbook of Mindfulness*, pp. 85–98, Edited by Fabrizio Didonna. New York: Springer Publisher.

Ladnier, R.D., and Massanari, A.E. (2000). Treating ADHD as Attachment Hyperactivity Disorder. In: *Handbook of Attachment Interventions*, pp. 27–65, Edited by Levy, P., USA: T.M. Academic Press.

Lama, D. (2000). A Journey to Happiness. In: *The Transformed Mind. Reflection on Truth, Love and Happiness*, pp. 23–49, Edited by Renuka Singh, Croydon: Coronet Paperback.

Music, G. (2015). Bringing up the Bodies: Psyche-soma, Body Awareness and Feeling at Ease. *British Journal of Psychotherapy*, Vol. 31(1): 4–12.

Music, R. (2014). Top Down and Bottom Up: Treating Triune, Executive Functioning, Emotional Regulation, the Brain and Child Psychotherapy. *Journal of Child Psychotherapy*, Vol. 40(1): 3–19.

Pally, R. (1997). How Brain Development is Shaped by Genetic and Environmental Factors: Development in Related Fields Neuroscience. *The International Journal of Psychoanalysis*, Vol. 78: 587–593.

Pally, R. (2000). *The Mind-Brain Relationship*. London & New York: Karnac Books.

Pozzi, M. (1993). The Use of Observation in the Psychoanalytic Treatment of a Twelve-Year-Old Boy with Asperger's Syndrome. *The International Journal of Psychoanalysis*, Vol. 84(5): 1333–1349.

Schore, A.N. (2001). Minds in the Making: Attachment, The Self-Organizing Brain, and Developmentally-Oriented Psychoanalytic Psychotherapy. *British Journal of Psychotherapy*, Vol. 17: 299–328.

Talge, N.M., Neal, C., Glover, V., and The Early Stress, Translational Research and Prevention Science Network: Fetal and Neonatal Experience on Child and Adolescent Mental Health. (2007). Antenatal Maternal Stress and Long-Term Effects on Child Neurodevelopment: How and Why? *Journal of Child Psychology and Psychiatry*, Vol. 48(3/4): 245–261.

Treadway, M.T., and Lazar, S.W. (2010). The Neurobiology of Mindfulness. In: *Clinical Handbook of Mindfulness*, pp. 45–57, Edited by Fabrizio Didonna. New York: Springer Publisher.

Wax, R. (2016). *A Mindfulness Guide for the Frazzled*. Penguin. (Wikipedia.org/zh-hk/File:1511_The_Limbic_Lobe.jpg)

4 Pregnancy

Like the ground turning green in a spring wind.
Like birdsong beginning inside the egg.
Like the universe coming into existence,
the lover wakes and whirls
in a dancing joy,
then kneels down
in praise.

Rumi, circa 2500, p. 275

The literature

Seneviratne and Conray (2004) write:

Not only do pregnancy and child birth exert important psychological and physiological effects on a woman's life but a mother's pregnancy and postnatal difficulties impact indelibly on her child and, reciprocally, the temperamental health and behavior of the child impact on the mother's well-being. The psychological fit between the two, in the context of the larger family, carries significant implications for both.

(p. 123)

Raphael-Leff (1991) recognised that within the specificity of each, individual pregnancy, there are a number of experiences, which are common to most pregnant mothers. First of all, she has to accept the idea and the reality of having to share the inner space of her body with a "genetically foreign body" (Ibid., p. 45). Then she has to tolerate that the "inexplorable doubts undermine her faith about her capacity to contain, sustain and preserve the precarious little embryo", wondering if her womb is spacious, safe and secure enough or narrow, poisonous and dangerous. The impermeability of internal barriers, as the author describes it, loosens the boundary between levels of consciousness and memory (Ibid., p. 49). Inevitably, mood swings, intense urges and moments of insight into one's unconscious may characterise this period. A pregnant woman is essentially alone as it is her body that changes; it is her emotional, hormonal and emotional states that are affected. "There may be a man around, even one who is keen to play the paternal role for the baby, but if he is unsuitable in her mind as a father, he adds to her burden of already having responsibly to map out her future child's life" (Ibid., p. 54). This clearly applied to my patient Sonia, as we will see in the vignette below. Raphael-Leff continues,

> Clearly, pregnancy can be utilized as a time of personal growth and emotional "rebirth", enriching the woman, fostering the integration of disparate parts of herself, her past and personality by re-incorporating facets of herself that have been split off, neglected or disowned.
>
> (Ibid., p. 52)

In order to achieve this, psychotherapeutic help may be needed. There is a growing evidence that that mother's emotional states affect the growing baby: for example, the production of the hormone cortisol, when under stress, passes through the placenta and affects the birth weight of the baby (Cleaver et al., 1999, p. 48). We also read that, with regard to making use of drugs or alcohol:

> The effect of drinking or drugs on the developing foetus is dependent on three interrelated factors: the pharmacological make-up of the drug, the gestation of pregnancy, and the route/amount of drug use. [...] The foetus is most susceptible to structural damage during 4–12 weeks of gestation; drugs taken later generally affect growth or cause neo-natal addiction.
>
> (Cleaver, H. et al., p. 49)

Moreover, it has been documented that "the negative behavior and attitudes of some drug-using women toward their children are in large part attributable to the accumulation of large numbers of stressors in the mothers' lives" (Hans, 2004, p. 206). My patient Sonia had used drugs and alcohol but was aware of the destructive effect they would have had on her baby, hence had stopped immediately when she realised she was pregnant.

Clinical vignette

Sonia, Larry and baby Regan

It was a risky pregnancy: Sonia had been using hard drugs on and off but had stopped once she had become pregnant. Yet, there had been grave concern about her unstable personality, which had required counselling since the age of twelve. Sonia was now a mother of three children aged eight and above and expecting her fourth child from her third partner. We met when she was three-months pregnant and felt anxious about this unplanned pregnancy, unwilling to terminate it, yet burdened at the prospect of going through it all for a fourth time. She had been friendly with the baby's father, Larry, for a number of years but when their relationship had become more intimate, she got pregnant with his baby. She hoped to be able to give this child a proper family with a father, which had not happened with her previous children. In this way, she may have a chance to repair some of her past damage.

Larry, for his part, was keen to have his first baby, but Sonia lost her positive feelings towards him and could not trust him to be an adequate father. She feared being let down and abandoned i.e. that the infant parts of herself would not find a nest in Larry. These were her life-long leitmotifs, having been neglected and not liked by her mother, squashed in between a few other siblings, and just about having survived thanks to her father's positive presence in her childhood. She reported that abandonment had been a big issue in her life and it had been the focus of much of her previous cognitive and other types of therapies.

Quite soon in our first meeting, she spoke of her current major preoccupation i.e. the sexual ill-treatment she had been the victim of, a few years earlier and which she proceeded to describe in detail. She was waiting for counselling for the PTSD she had developed since then, but was keen to start working with me regarding her baby-in-the womb. The latter she had ignored a great deal and was indeed struck by my comment that – in her mind – the baby was not Larry's baby but was the abuser's baby. So much was the intensity of that still-unprocessed experience that she confused or fused the bad violent past with the current, creative intercourse. This seemed to clarify both the denial of a growing life inside her and the ambivalence about wanting it.

She felt relieved as she had wanted a fourth child in the past but this had now been clouded by that traumatic experience. Eventually, she decided to keep the pregnancy and worked as best as possible to make it good. She knew she was a good mum and had done well with her other three children who, according to her, had rescued her from depression and episodes of acting out. They had given her a good reason to be mature, she once said to me. However, her self-esteem was up and down and when she said she had enjoyed meeting me after our first session and I replied that I too had enjoyed meeting her, she said: "You may not say so after five sessions". We had agreed to meet five times to begin with, then to review the work.

We explored both hers and Larry's background and their current relationship to make the remaining six months in the womb as comfortable as possible "for the little sod", as Sonia would call him affectionately, and in her words "in line with my family tradition". She was well aware that her anxious, agitated state was not conducive to her pregnancy, but was not able to be different, she said. Her great agitation and her relentless, incessant pouring out of negative and devaluing comments about Larry, which I verbalised at different moments, but to no avail, needed a different technique. Whatever I was saying, doing or how I was being would not stop her. She needed to pass on some of the violence and badness she had herself suffered from.

I decided to introduce simple mindful exercises, which she soon accepted and practiced eagerly with me to begin with. So, we began breathing together slowly, feeling and observing the breath going in and coming out of the nostrils and also focusing on bodily sensations and imagining the baby inside her. Sonia began to be able to both feel the baby, to gradually follow his movements inside her, thinking of him growing and swimming in her womb. Eventually, things calmed down and the change in her attitude and style of communication became palpable in sessions: she spoke more calmly, observed herself, refrained from blaming Larry and others and took more responsibilities for her way of being.

Sonia had high hopes for this pregnancy, since her previous ones had been coloured with post-natal depression, violence and abuse. She wanted a proper family life with Larry and their first year of life together boded well. But things changed after that first year and she became disappointed with him. In sessions with them both, evidence mounted that she was projecting onto him a lot of her earlier life disappointments: to me he appeared to be a good-enough partner, to her he was like a disappointing mother.

Larry was a likely candidate for Sonia's attacks and rejections. He had been rejected by his violent and abusive parents and sent to live elsewhere. He was also a substance user. There was an unconscious fit between them (Balint, 1993). His domineering mother was similar to Sonia's own and Sonia's depression made her feel like her own passive and absent mother, whom Sonia wanted to be better than.

Both Sonia and Larry were soon to be evicted from their respective homes and were negotiating re-housing with the Council. However, while Sonia could be pro-active, well organised, able to get help from friends and local services, Larry was more dependent, helpless and somewhat restricted in creating good options for his life. He did not accept individual therapy for himself, however he often came to our joint sessions and benefitted from them.

The summer holiday – four months after we began – destabilised our work. Sonia cancelled sessions, avoided me and openly rejected my attempt to link up with her; however, when we eventually met, she agreed that she needed to see me more often. However, she had to take total control and when I changed one session, she cancelled several. She left me one month before stopping for the summer holiday. Her baby was due then but we could only speak on the phone and not meet.

She sounded distant, but well organised and had been re-housed. The day after the baby's birth, she returned my call, while still in hospital, to inform me that all went well. Larry was helping and her older children were keen to see her back home with baby Regan. She was just tired and could not commit to coming to the Centre as yet. However, only two weeks later she came to see me with baby Regan. She was pleased and told me of his quick birth and that she was back to her old self. She noticed the continuity between when he was in the womb and after he was born: he was feeding every two hours.

She felt her depression coming back and started medication, remembering how hard the pregnancy had been without antidepressants but also feeling proud of having made it. She was warm and affectionate with baby Regan, although at times a little rough. I verbalised this and she was able to take it on board well, without feeling persecuted or criticised. We practiced mindfulness together and this helped her to see him as a baby-baby and not as a baby-sod.

Our work continued for another year and a half at her home with Larry visiting and feeling proud of his first baby. She had grown more comfortable with his care of Regan and trusted him to look after him even overnight. When she felt established enough in herself and within her family, she was happy to say goodbye to me and − as she said − for me to give my help to other needy families.

I contacted her again about three years later, at the time of writing about our psychotherapy work and was fortunate to be able to meet her and the whole family at their home. It was an improvised visit after attempted telephone calls and Sonia was very pleased to see me again. She talked a lot about the latest events. Larry arrived from work, joined us briefly and updated me a little on his current life, while Ragan was extremely excited and in no time, was sitting comfortably on my knees, chatting non-stop as if he had always known me. Soon he wiggled away to prance around but did respond to Sonia's limit-setting. In a few months he was going to start a new nursery closer to their home and which he had already visited. Sonia was doing well, was working part-time in a local pub and had managed to stay off drugs and drinks ever since our work. She had some brief counselling for her past traumas and was awaiting deeper psychotherapy, she said. She read this piece very attentively and smiled benevolently at being reminded of those days. We parted warmly.

Bibliography

Balint, E. (1993). *Before I Was I: Psychoanalysis and the Imagination*, Edited by J. Mitchell and M. Parsons, London: Free Association Books.

Cleaver, H., Unell, I., and Aldgate, J. (1999). Child development and parenting capacity. In: *Children's Needs -Parenting Capacity. The impact of parental mental illness, problem alcohol and drug use, and domestic violence on children's development.* London: The Stationary Office.

Hans, S.L. (2004). When Mothers Abuse Drugs. In: *Parental Psychiatric Disorder*, pp. 203–216. Second edition. Edited by Gopfert, M., Webster, J., and Seeman, M.V., Cambridge: Cambridge University Press.

Raphael-Leff, J. (1991). *Psychological Processes of Childbearing*. London: Chapman and Hall.

Rumi. (circa 1250). Birdsong from Inside the Egg. In: *The Essential Rumi*, Translated by Barks, C. with Moyne, J. (1995). pp. 274–275. London: Penguin Books.

Seneviratne, G., and Conray, S. (2004). Perinatal Mental Illness: Nature/Nurture. In: *Parental Psychiatric Disorder*, pp. 123–138. Second edition. Edited by Gopfert, M., Webster, J., and Seeman, M.V., Cambridge: Cambridge University Press.

5   From unbearable, persecutory guilt to tolerable, reparative guilt in working with severely damaged babies and their parents

"Ask," said he,
"With humble heart, that he unbar the bolt."
Piously at his holy feet devolved
I cast me, praying him for pity's sake
That he would open to me; but first fell
Thrice on my bosom prostrate.
                    Dante Canto IX vv 96–101

The literature

Klein wrote:

> The baby's first object of love and hate – his mother – is both desired
> and hated with all the intensity and strength that is characteristic of the
> early urges of the baby. In the very beginning he loved his mother at the
> time that she is satisfying his needs for nourishment, alleviating his feel-
> ings of hunger and giving him the sensual pleasure which he experiences
> when his mouth is stimulated by sucking at her breast. [...]. But when
> the baby is hungry and his desires are not gratified, or when he is feeling
> bodily pain or discomfort, then the whole situation suddenly alters.
> Hatred and aggressive feelings are aroused and he becomes dominated
> by the impulses to destroy the very person who is the object of all his
> desires and who in his mind is linked up with everything he experi-
> ences – good and bad alike.
>
> (Klein, 1937, pp. 306–7)

She continues:

> This leads to feelings of guilt and again to wishes to make good: a mixture
> of feelings which has an important bearing not only on our relations with
> brothers and sisters but, since relations to people in general are modelled

on the same pattern, also on our social attitude and on feelings of love and guilt and the wish to make good in later life.

(Ibid., p. 310)

However, feelings of guilt "if they are too great, have the effect of inhibiting productive activities and interests". (Ibid., pp. 335–6).

Hinshelwood (1989) writes that guilt in its earlier and more primitive form is of a persecutory and retaliatory nature and the infant's ego is felt under threat of death by harsh punishment (p. 314). While the more evolved type of guilt allows for a deep sense of regret and of responsibility for the hurt or damage caused to the other and a wish to make things better. The above-mentioned authors alert us to feelings of guilt as they originate in infancy.

In this chapter, I focus mainly on parental guilt and how this can be transformed from its more crude, persecutory form to a more benevolent and reparatory guilt vis-à-vis one's own baby.

Clinical vignettes

Eva and baby Martha

Baby Martha, aged nine months, and her mother Eva, were referred to our parent-infant service by Eva's psychiatrist, concerned about the effect on the baby, of the mother's depression and Obsessional Compulsive Disorder, for which Eva was being treated. A family history of mental illness was also present as Eva's deceased mother had been diagnosed with schizophrenia: Eva remembered looking after her and feeling ashamed when her friends went to her home and her mum was speaking incoherently. Eva's mother had died of cancer when she was about 12 years old and Eva was then brought up by an aunt, who had helped her with the first three children but was now dead and could not assist her with Martha. Eva hardly met her father although her children's father was around and helpful but no longer her partner. Men have not provided her with much emotional support.

Martha had been admitted to the intensive care unit of a large children's hospital at the age of six months for pneumonia, severe lung necrosis and again, a month before we met, as they had found bubbles on her lungs and needed to suck them out. Martha was the fourth child – after an eleven-year-old girl and seven-year-old twins – of a separated mother, whose life had been ridden with adversities and losses. Eva had not managed to mourn her many losses, but developed OCD at the time of her beloved aunt's death. Eva felt guilty and ashamed about her OCD and her panic attacks. She feared damaging her children and was overconcerned about not washing the fruit and vegetables well enough nor cooking the food long enough! She felt inadequate as a mother and was ridden with guilt particularly about Martha's unfortunate illness and felt that Martha was closer to her older sister than to herself.

She clung to Martha especially after Martha became ill, was overprotective and was too anxious to let her grow freely. When we first met, she was still breastfeeding her and let her have access to her breast whenever she wanted with no rules or timing: this contributed to Martha becoming rather tyrannical. She was described as always getting her way, and the whole family revolved around her pitilessly. Eva could not feel much sadness nor cry over losing people or her home country: she said she wanted to leave everything behind and move on with her life. However, when Eva was in hospital with Martha for a long time and the family had to give away their dear, little dog as no one could look after him, Eva cried profusely. Perhaps it was safer to attach to the healthy dog she had had for many years and even before Martha's birth, than to a sickly baby. Interestingly, Martha, too, never cried – she only had excessive mucus in her lungs – and even the hospital doctors were very surprised. I wondered if her lungs were somehow crying and producing excessive mucus or "solid tears", which could not be absorbed by Martha's little body. Eva listened to this idea with no reaction.

In these first sessions, we were sitting on the floor on a padded mat with baby toys, but Martha was not to play with them, nor put them in her mouth, in case she choked or got infected. Eva could not even let Martha explore a toy and every time she wobbled, Mum pounced anxiously on her and grabbed her. I addressed them both by saying: "Oh dear, you nearly toppled over and Mum got very, very worried in case you fell and hurt yourself and she caught you!" Eva responded with a knowing smile. We spoke of creating an extra impediment for Martha by being overprotective of her and I encouraged Eva to let her explore those safe toys freely: she revealed that she always feared Martha would die.

Gradually more freedom to play was given to her and she took to the egg toy and liked to push – with great energy – the chicks into their opened eggs to make them squeak. She expressed a lot of aggression in banging the eggs and squashing the chicks, possibly her pent-up anger; I observed her and described her play and gave words to her feelings.

Eva spent most of the sessions recollecting her anxious, obsessional thoughts about the dog they had to give away, her dead auntie, Martha's breathing, and the incapacity to set healthy and necessary limits on her tyrannical demands. Her loneliness was also a feature of our work: although Eva had good friends, she could not talk to them intimately as they would not understand her obsessive churning over everything.

Mindfulness seemed very appropriate in this situation, where breathing was somewhat impaired and learning to direct and observe the breath and her bodily sensations may be of great benefit to Eva; it would help her direct her attention to something else than her thoughts. It would also affect Martha indirectly. Eva had to practice this with me and observe the effect on her baby, especially when Martha was fretful and restless. In sessions, we noticed that Martha slowed down and could focus on toys for a little longer. Eva reported also practicing mindfulness at night when she was anxious and could not sleep: it calmed her down greatly.

Martha, now twelve months old, was still not teething and holding onto breastfeeding on demand. Mum did not feel ready to wean her off as yet, she said, hoping to receive my approval. Separations from the breast as well as from sessions were difficult and a painful reminder of her past losses. Eva would "leave" me before the term was over and was frozen on our return. It was difficult to help her grieve and to let go of her obsessions: we understood that her real friends were her churning thoughts: always there protecting her from sorrow, anger and frustration, therefore, she also could not help Martha let go of the breast. In line with this state of mind, she admitted that when her older children were not at home or with her, she always worried that something tragic might happen to them – similarly to what had just happened to Martha's father's nephew's son, who had been recently killed in a car accident abroad.

In sessions, Eva started to engage more with Martha and they had some playful moments together; she also let Martha be more independent and allow her developmental trajectory to be resumed. Martha began eating a few bits of solid food and this would slowly lead to a noticeable reduction in her demand for the breast. Her lungs improved but not completely and she still needed occasional hospital check-ups and to have the mucus cleared. She also started to become angry when she was not allowed something: she would screech, throw things and be bossy and tyrannical to the point that it was almost impossible not to give into her. Eventually, Eva admitted that she, herself, was the problem: she was afraid of damaging Martha and making her ill, if she made her cry by withholding her breast; she would feel like a bad mother. Also crying was a charged issue for Eva: no mother had been there for her in her early life, to help her manage tears and distress. She realised that she would feel too sad at taking the breast away from Martha and I wonder whether she was keen to give her what she, herself, had not been given by her ill mother.

The shadow of Martha's illness was still widespread around the family and they all tended to give into the littlest one out of fear and guilt. However, some progress occurred and Eva proposed to cut back on our sessions but trying to reduce the frequency was difficult and once we had a two months' break, Eva regressed badly in her obsessional thinking, anguished feelings about her own death and suffered from intense panic attacks. This inevitable, uneven course of therapy was soon contained and we met again. Martha was growing into a curious, inquisitive, and mobile little girl going from all fours to her two feet, but still determined to either have her mother's breast or else hardly any other food! Martha's father also showed up to a couple of sessions to talk over his recent loss of a family member and Eva livened up and became happier both about herself and with Martha. Eva's churning thoughts diminished almost entirely and her anguish about the lost dog relented its grip on her: she was on the path to healing.

I had the chance to meet all her children during a half-term holiday and subsequent home visits: they were delightful, healthy, ordinary kids, doing well at school, with friends and able to enjoy their lives: Eva had indeed manged very well with them. Eva's intense and persecuting guilt also decreased and the relationship with Martha became healthier and growth-promoting, no longer life-stifling. By the end of our work, which lasted a year and a half, Martha was a happy, inquisitive and mischievous little girl, who played freely and was engaged with people and her surroundings. Mum's panic attacks at night and during the day still occurred but were now managed by mindfulness and breathing techniques. The ongoing psychodynamic parent-infant psychotherapy aided by mindfulness practice had offered Eva maternal understanding and containment of her deprived childhood experiences and paternal-type structure and boundaries, which had led to good resilience and more self-esteem.

I met Eva, Martha and the rest of the family, again three years later on the occasion of writing this piece for the book as I wanted to show it to Eva. She smiled and stopped at the point that described Martha as being bossy and said she was still bossy, telling people what to do, to play with her etc.! Eva was feeling better about herself and was now enjoying cooking again for the family. We went to pick up Martha and the boys from nursery and school and walked back home together. Martha kept looking at me with curiosity and – once back home – sat close to me on the settee to show me her school books. She spoke English with me and Polish with her mum fluently. They were grateful for this visit and we parted somewhat sadly.

Leila and baby Oliver

Oliver, aged nine months, and his mother Leila came to our Service on the advice of their health visitor. Leila, after having managed valiantly the risky pregnancy and birth of a premature and physically damaged baby, had suddenly lost all her confidence in caring for Oliver. She described being gripped with anxiety, when left alone with Oliver, especially when it came to feeding time. She also referred to her inability to manage the baby, when he was occasionally sick and of getting sick herself; then having to turn to her own family for help. Oliver's weight was very low but when he started on solids and the high calorific milk recommended by the dietician, he began putting on weight and enjoying his feedings. Nevertheless, his devoted mother continued feeling anxious and overstressed at feeding time. Oliver was described as a delightful and happy baby with good attachment to his mother, bur developmentally behind for his age.

At the beginning of our work, undertaken together with a colleague, Oliver, "deposited" by his mother on the big cushion on the floor mat, lay very still, motionless, almost paralysed, looking lifeless, while mother began her story in a somewhat uncertain way, this being her first counselling experience. The pregnancy had been fraught with Leila's health issues, till she – intuitively – took herself to the hospital, where she was admitted as a matter of urgency and given a Caesarean Section. Oliver had stopped breathing in the womb. He was resuscitated immediately and kept, together with his mother, in the special care unit for several days. This was six weeks before the due date. Although Leila agreed that she had saved her baby's life, she still felt negative about everything. She said she had felt devastated especially in view of the fact that she had never wanted to have a baby but had conceded to external pressure. She felt she had been punished for that, yet she was able to look at that bundle on the cushion, lovingly and with a mixture of sadness, regret and guilt.

After hearing of this difficult story and in view of Oliver's earlier breathing difficulties and Leila's anxieties, it felt appropriate to introduce mindful breathing. This could help her focus her mind on her breathing in an attempt to divert her from her negative churning and overthinking. We suggested that she observe her slow breathing while holding Oliver in her arms. She seemed interested in trying it at home, too, and reported some temporary benefits and having a calmer mind.

During one session, it was noticed that Leila played with Oliver by throwing a blanket over his face and removing it after what felt to us too-long a time. Leila repeated this game several times with no awareness of its impact on her baby, who looked taken aback, puzzled and struggled to push the blanket off his face. However, baby Oliver soon gave a faint smile and then did the same to himself by covering his face, then moving the blanket away. Was mother unconsciously playing out her hostility towards her baby? Was she projecting her own feeling of being smothered by her baby? Was Oliver already adapting to his mother's game by smiling then copying his mother and identifying with the aggressor? (Fraiberg et al., 1975). The feeling of alarm and the anxiety were experienced only by us two therapists. We were able to address this in a light way, which Leila could take on, to some degree, and she gave up playing it. However, her ambivalence showed up again when she gave him the needed dummy by holding it too far away from him somewhat tantalising him, and he could not reach it. Leila also would address Oliver as "the baby" and not by his name. In keeping this safe distance, she seemed to protect herself in case Oliver became ill again and died.

Leila had accepted our offer of five sessions and a review of the progress. From the third session onward, the progress was constant, and Leila was trying hard to become a better mother. She stopped giving her baby to family people as soon as there was a small hiccup or a stressful moment at home. She told us that she had thought of what we would have said and her mother would have done and she, herself, managed to do it, without having to call upon her mother. Oliver would calm down almost immediately and "magically", she said. This new process of separation from her own mother and internalisation of our thinking had begun. Leila was no longer keen to have to return to work: she was feeling happier, more confident and enjoyed being a mother.

Oliver, for his part, was now feeding well and looking at his mother's eyes more openly. During a moment of play with Leila, now sitting comfortably enough on the floor mat next to Oliver and us too, Oliver dropped a soft cube from his hand. He looked momentarily puzzled, taken aback, a little shocked. Leila gave it back to him and he smiled broadly at having the precious object back in his grip. Leila noticed all this herself and was surprised. I described this game to Oliver with an emphatic tone and baby talk (and to mum indirectly) and linked Oliver's reaction to his age, when babies feel the separation from their mothers acutely.

So far, we had not detected any obvious resistance or guilt in Leila, who had been appreciative of our understanding and had also been surprised to hear this information, which was new to her, about separation anxiety. However, pretty soon, she began to feel bad about having planned a week holiday without the baby and even wondered if she would have to cancel the trip. Our work was now aiming at containing her guilt, which was increased by her imminent return to long hours of work and the plan to hand over Oliver to a nanny. We worked on her negative transference towards us, the bad therapists, who had introduced her to such painful knowledge, but she had not overtly responded to it.

Her guilt had the quality of a real persecution, which was hard to temperate and come to terms with. We made plans that would fit with her working schedule and would allow us to monitor the progress and Oliver's adjustment to the nanny. Leila agreed to continue seeing us on two further occasions but eventually cancelled those sessions. We felt that her guilt had taken over and she dared not return to us for fear that we would have made her feel even worse. Perhaps by cancelling those sessions she was unconsciously and concretely agreeing with our hypothesis that we were bad people, who were causing her suffering; hence it was better to stay away and just make the best of the improvement achieved. She had, in fact, been aware and acknowledged the help received in those few sessions.

Perhaps Oliver's failure to thrive had been partly influenced by his mother's intense ambivalence and aversion towards this unwanted, sickly and damaged baby. Through our psychoanalytic psychotherapeutic work some good progress had been achieved but more work would have been useful in order to consolidate the mother-baby relationship and contain the mother's guilt more deeply. However, this did not happen, probably due to Leila's fear of her unacknowledged and unbearable guilt. We learnt that the family moved out of the area, rendering any possible, further contact untenable.

Bibliography

Alighieri, D. (1265–1321). The Divine Comedy. *Canto IX*, Vol. vv: 96–101. The Harvard Classics. 1909–14.

Fraiberg, S., Adelson, E., and Shapiro, V. (1975). Ghosts in the Nursery. *Journal of the American Academy of Child Psychiatry*, Vol. 14: 387–421.

Hinshelwood, R.D. (1989). *A Dictionary of Kleinian Thoughts*. London: Free Association Books.

Klein, M. (1937). *Love, Guilt and Reparation and Other Works*, pp. 306–343. London: The Hogarth Press. 1975.

6   Immigration, dislocation and loss

I alone am inert, like a child that has not yet given sign;
Like an infant that has not yet smiled.
I droop and drift, as though I belonged nowhere.
All men have enough and to spare;
I alone seem to have lost everything.
[...] I alone am dark.
[...] I alone, depressed.
I seem unsettled as the ocean;
Blown adrift, never brought to a stop.
[...] I prize no sustenance that comes not from the Mother's breast.

Lao Tzŭ, XX pp. 136–7

The literature

Freud (1917) writes,

> Mourning is regularly the reaction to the loss of a loved person, or to the
> loss of some abstraction which has taken the place of one, such as one's
> country, liberty, an ideal, and so on. In some people the same influences
> produce melancholia instead of mourning and we consequently suspect
> them of a pathological disposition.
>
> (p. 243)

Further on we read,

> Reality-testing has shown that the loved one no longer exists, and it pro-
> ceeds to demand that all libido shall be withdrawn from its attachments to
> that object. This demand arouses understandable opposition – it is a matter
> of general observation that people never willingly abandon a libidinal pos-
> ition, not even, indeed, when a substitute is already beckoning to them.
>
> (p. 244)

In the normal mourning process "the withdrawal of the libido from [the] object and a displacement of it onto a new one, but something different", takes place. This means that in mourning, the main task is to acknowledge what has happened, accept it emotionally and sort out the many, ambivalent feelings, lost hopes, expectations and thoughts, so that the memory of the lost object is put into perspective, both allowing life to continue and even to enhance it.

> The distinguishing mental features of melancholia are a profoundly painful dejection, cessation of interest in the outside world, loss of the capacity to love, inhibition of all activity, and a lowering of the self-regarding feeling to the degree that finds utterance in self-reproaches and self-revilings, and culminates in a delusional expectation of punishment.
>
> (p. 244)

Freud continues,

> Each single one of the memories and expectations in which the libido is bound to the object is brought up and hypercathected, and detachment of the libido is accomplished in respect of it [...and] when the work of mourning is completed the ego becomes free and uninhibited again. [...] melancholia is in some way related to an object-loss which is withdrawn from consciousness, in contradistinction to mourning, in which there is nothing about the loss that is unconscious.
>
> (p. 245)

Klein (1929) observed and studied depression in children and like Freud "she knew that guilt and depression had to do with losing and mourning an ambivalently loved object" (Hinshelwood, 1991, pp. 138–9). We read about her little patient Erna, aged six when she began treatment due to her severe obsessional neuroses with hidden paranoia;

> who often made me to be a child, while she was the mother or the teacher. I then had to undergo fantastic tortures and humiliation. [...] After her sadism had spent itself in these fantasies, apparently unchecked by any inhibition, (all this came about after we had done a good deal of analysis), reaction would set in in the form of deep depression, anxiety and bodily exhaustion. Her play then reflected her incapacity to bear this tremendous oppression, which manifested itself in a number of serious symptoms.
>
> (Klein, Ibid., pp. 199–200)

In her 1935 paper Klein writes that in the first few months of the baby's life,

> the ego feels itself constantly menaced in its possession of internalized good objects. It is full of anxiety lest such objects should die. Both in children and adults suffering from depression, I have discovered the

dread of harbouring dying or dead objects (especially the parents) inside one and an identification of the ego with objects in this condition. From the very beginning of psychic development there is a constant correlation of real objects with those installed within the ego. It is for this reason that the anxiety which I have just described manifests itself in a child's exaggerated fixation to his mother or whoever looks after it. [...] The absence of the mother arouses in the child anxiety lest it should be handed over to bad objects, external and internalized, either because of her *death* or because of her return in the guise of a *"bad"* mother.

(p. 266)

The authors Bourne and Lewis (1984), who studied perinatal miscarriages and losses, write:

For normal mourning it is necessary to hold images of the dead person, internalised in the mind's inner world until, eventually, there is resolution, relinquishment. In mourning, the dual processes of "taking in" the loss and eventually freeing oneself from clinging to the past, "letting go", could both interfere with the vaguely similar yet vitally different state of mind [...] required during pregnancy to cherish the idea of the new baby, actually inside the mother's body. The baby will seem to be endangered by bad feelings and frightening ideas, inevitable in the mourning process.

(p. 32)

And further below: "Children born after a bereavement are at risk of becoming 'replacement children' [...]. Infancy and childhood are affected by the parents' anxieties and depression, together with their confused wishes and expectations carried over from unresolved mourning" (p. 32). "When mourning is interrupted by pregnancy, anticipation of later difficulty will prepare for unfinished grieving, postponed until the baby is safely in existence. Effective mourning may then be possible, when psychotherapy may also be timely" (p. 33). Lewis (1979) writes:

Reasons why pregnancy interrupts mourning are complex. Normal parenting entails mixed feelings even for the most wanted baby. There are comparable mixed feelings for the dead person, however loved, that mourning helps. During mourning the dead person is consciously imagined as being taken inside our minds and our bodies. The dazed mourner will say, "I can't take it in yet." The dead can be unconsciously felt dead yet active inside us; imagined variously as alive and supportive or as damaged, burdensome, or persecuting. The dead person and the live fetus both inhabit the mother's body and mind. Because a pregnant mother's idea of her fetus is inevitably imaginary and poorly defined she can easily confuse her unconscious mixed feelings for the fetus with those for the dead. It protects her fetus from the dangerous summation of her confused mixed feelings if she blocks the process of mourning.

(p. 27)

Another text, which is relevant to my work with the first family described here below, is by Renos Papadopoulos, editor of the book, *Therapeutic Care for Refugees: No Place Like Home* (2002). He writes about the meaning of home, and the sense of dislocation that can occur for refugees where the physical and emotional landscape of what home signifies become re-configured, often in devastating ways: "Whenever the home is lost, all the organizing and containing functions break wide open and there is a possibility of disintegration at all three levels: at the individual-personal level; at the family-marital level; and at the socio-economic/cultural-political level" (p. 24). He goes on to elucidate on the connections between home and containment:

> ... family stories express the interconnections between the personal, family and wider parameters within the context of a sense of home that enables the holding and containing of all opposite and contradictory elements that threaten to disrupt the sense of continuity and predictability. It is this very continuity that is disrupted when people lose their homes and become refugees.
>
> (pp. 25–6)

I have quoted extensively from Freud, Klein, Bourne, Lewis and Papadopoulos as my work with Josephina and her baby Emma was almost a test-book description of the thinking of these authors and clinicians.

Clinical vignettes

Josephine and baby Emma

As mentioned, we will see in this case history all the points made by the above authors: Mum's move from her conscious memories and longing for her deceased three-year-old son, to unconscious, repressed feelings about her own country, which she was not allowed to visit due to poor immigration advice she'd received. All this propelled her into a state of delayed melancholia after the birth of her second baby since the death of her son, but not after the birth of her first one. Compounded with the loss of her son, the impossibility of visiting her family in her country of origin, magnified her sense of dislocation and grief leading her into a state of deep depression. At that point, Emma aged four months, was referred by the health visitor concerned about her mother having become particularly sad and tearful and being unclear whether this was a sign of post-natal depression and of its impact on the newborn baby girl.

Josephine came with her three daughters for an after-school appointment to the Children Centre, where we first met. She had chosen this time for practical reasons, she said but, with hindsight, I think this gave her the opportunity to come with her children, who were to shield her from an unknown and anxious situation. She was not sure why her health visitor had referred her, even though she had agreed to the referral in view of her recent outbursts of sadness and tearfulness. Soon the story unfolded in an unending flood of tears as she recounted the events of her child's death. A few years earlier their little boy aged three died accidentally by choking on food and despite his mother's prompt and determined care and attempt to save him. "It was too late, when half-an-hour after the event, the ambulance arrived" she said. The family was devastated and entered a period of grief and mourning, which was still going on three years later and was most acute on anniversary dates. However, Josephine became pregnant almost immediately, well-aware that she was eager to replace the dead child, although she later realised that nothing could ever replace him. That pregnancy was fraught with anxieties and fears that something equally tragic might happen and when things went well, the whole family rejoiced. A baby girl was born and despite mother and older daughter's incessant grieving – father was around and very supportive but not mentioned much – the new baby grew, apparently healthy, and at that time was without any developmental delay. However, Josephine's unresolved grief compounded by real and unjust issues regarding their status as immigrants, erupted when Emma was born and again at the approaching anniversary of her boy's death.

In the first session, baby Emma was being given to the older daughter and looked like a rag doll, not floppy but very still, cringing a lot and looking alert. When the older daughter eventually returned Emma to Mum, she placed her on her legs to get ready to breastfeed her. I cringed as I saw that motionless bundle, who could easily roll over mum's legs and fall on the floor. But Josephine was confident and already experienced with her other babies, so nothing untoward happened and Emma lay still and motionless, waiting to be fed. Something similar happened by the end of the session but I was by then more used to that and more confident that Emma would not be dropped. At the breast, she sucked for only a few minutes then fell asleep and so remained till the end of this painful session.

Josephine agreed to meet without the girls the following week, but sessions were cancelled, and the anniversary came and went without us meeting again for a long spell of time. We had some contact via telephone and her ambivalence was expressed openly: she did not want to talk, think or remember as this would have made her sad for a long time after. Yet, as I would witness, once home visits were arranged, thoughts about the dead boy, the events that led to his death, her enormous guilt, feeling of regret and unforgiveness were constantly on her mind, almost like an obsession, which would not leave her day or night. Uncountable photographs of her dead child were scattered in all corners of their home: many more than photos of the living children. Sessions at the Children Centre alternated with sessions in the family kitchen, when mother was too depressed or busy to come to the nearby children centre.

Most of my work with Josephine unfolded around her deeply persecutory guilt and unforgiveness for the death of her little boy: we went over and over, again and again, the traumatic events and her wish that she could have done something different and saved him. If only she could reverse time and history! Unanswerable questions were uttered repeatedly, contradictory feelings and accusations towards both herself and others poured out of her pained heart: "Why me? I am a good mother! Perhaps I did not look after him enough. It was my punishment, but for what? The ambulance did not come fast enough!" Her relentless guilt was now paralysing her interaction with Emma, who complied dutifully by being quiet and undemanding. There was nothing Josephina could do to be different, or to feel different, she said, meaning that nothing would have brought the little boy back to life.

Everything in her life was spoilt and she could not enjoy much of her three other children; she just wanted to go back to her country, to her roots as everything in this country was a reminder of her loss. At first, I was of no help to her but just a reminder of unbearably painful losses. However, I persevered and continued offering to see her and Emma, without pressurising her, and listened patiently and processed her difficult issues emotionally.

During those first months of work, Josephine had little emotional space for baby Emma, who was often restless, fretful, a poor sleeper and looked very serious, like a little old woman. When Josephine in tears breastfed Emma, she always had her dead son in mind not the alive, suckling infant in her lap. Amongst copious tears, she once revealed her anxious phantasy of having "killed" her little boy by not having saved him. Emma would move her legs and feet restlessly and almost mirrored her mum's sad movement. She never slept well or long enough, only napped and also tended to be constipated. My thoughts went to this baby, whose sleep could only bring her little peace or rest, and whose emotions could not flow smoothly out of her little body but instead came in jerky moves or remained trapped inside. Had she rested well, she might have reminded her mum of the dead boy. For a whole year Josephine had cried, never gone out but when the anniversary came again, family life stopped almost entirely, and they all went to the grave.

At a point of feeling hopeless and with no resource to offer her, I introduced mindfulness as a way to contain Josephine's relentless distress and to help focus her mind and breathing on both her bodily sensations and on Emma, rather than on her thoughts. In her situation she needed not to let her mind wonder incessantly to the loss of her dead, little boy but to rein it in and re-direct it to both her body and her alive baby. She did use it, and this contributed to her getting hold of her tortured thoughts and to calming down her mind.

Eventually the other painful problem emerged: Josephine was longing to go back to her country of origin to visit her family, whom she had not seen for many years and long before the boy's death. She was not allowed by the immigration system due to rather unsubstantial reasons related to her original entry into this country, many years earlier, and under a different name. Therefore, her grievance and feeling of loss and longing were compounded and directed to both her little boy and her country. I had to listen to her endless self-reproaches and blamings, doubts, regrets and to witness her intense and persecutory guilt, now directed mostly at the immigration situation.

In the end, and with an attentive and compassionate interest, gentle challenging on my part as well as her working through her losses and using mindfulness, too, changes began to occur. Josephine gradually began to play with Emma, offering her toys and rattles and interacting in a livelier way, and not just sticking her to her breast, plunking her on the mat or in her cot. She had turned a corner and was able to recognise it openly: she was less burdened by a tragedy, which will never be forgotten but had become tolerable and more acceptable.

Fifteen months later I was still in touch with the family and we could gradually face the end of our work: she could manage the feelings and memories about that tragic loss, which were inevitably stirred up by the final phase of our work. Being given the possibility to contact me again in the future, gave her a new experience of loss: this separation from me was not a death. She did send me a Christmas text message several months later, wishing me a happy festive time and sounding well enough herself.

Three years later I had the good fortune to meet Josephine, Emma and the other older girls again as I wanted to show her this writing. They were all well and Emma was described by her mum, as "still being bossy" but well settled at nursery and waiting to start preschool in a few months. Emma sat on the settee, close to her mum and looked shyly at me, then asked her mum for chips and ate them at the kitchen table, while watching television. Josephine was manging her family warmly and competently and was also going out more with friends and helping the less fortunate ones. Although she was more at peace with their tragic loss, she still wondered "why me? I am a good mother and always did and do my best!" This deep wound will always be there but in a way that fostered understanding and generosity in Josephine and in her family.

Becky and baby Max

Becky only came once with her four-month-old baby boy as she wanted to process "the many wrongs", that had occurred during and soon after her pregnancy. A professional woman, she had prepared everything in a perfect and ideal way, after having suffered several earlier miscarriages. She wanted to make sure that this pregnancy, birth and afterbirth would go well. However, events and situations went terribly wrong, but she did manage to preserve her relationship with baby Max and bonded well with him. "Yes, those many losses" had occurred both in her family life during her sick pregnancy and during the traumatic and life-threatening birth, leading to an internal collapse. She had lost the ideal baby and the ideal mother-father-baby relationship she had envisaged. Grieving seemed impossible as the gap between an idealised and a real outcome had been too wide. She became negative about her ability to be a mother; about her envied, "privileged" but also helpful partner and despondent about the real unavailable help from her extended family. Her general well-being had been disrupted by all those "wrongs" and she had thoughts and phantasies of how to end her life, but not that of her baby. Her nights were very bad, despite Max feeding and sleeping exceedingly well and deeply for long stretches of time. Becky had already tried mindfulness but to no avail. However, she accepted my suggestion to try walking mindfulness and thought it might help.

In our only session, baby Max sucked the bottle – alas not the breast as Becky would have dearly wished – then he regurgitated profusely. Becky was irreparably disappointed and longed to get out of this "cage" by returning to work quite soon and leaving baby Max in a nanny's care. She also left him in my temporary care in the session, when she suddenly leapt up, plonked him on the mat and went out to the nearby toilet. I was left feeling anxious about her fast plan to leave him and return to work. I must have put my foot "wrong", when Becky, concerned about affecting him with her state of mind, prompted me to confirm that babies are sensitive to mothers' states of mind, rather than me being able to understand and contain her anxiety.

By the end of this session, she felt she had been helped and wanted to come back, However, things turned "wrong" once she had left. Real circumstances went wrong on my part: I had written the wrong time on my diary plus my car going "wrong" and making me too late for our next session. A further internal loss of trust – this time trust in me – occurred. She felt betrayed, lost and cut off contact with me and our now-turned-wrong service, despite my many attempts to repair the "wrong". No chance to put things right was possible and I had to carry all the wrong, bad feelings, guilt and sadness. Grieving had been avoided, instead an abortion or murder of our newborn link took place, indeed, and mindfulness ... also failed!

In these unfortunate but rare circumstances, I always hope that the patient's acting out the "wrongness" and the therapist's perceived betrayal by cutting contact with the therapist, may preserve, at least to some extent, the relationship with the infant (Pozzi, 2011). If this does occur, it can provide temporary relief to the parent, shield the infant for the time being and offer a new experience of non-retaliation, although it is clearly not the best or healthiest way to manage psychic pain, to grow emotionally and to end treatment.

Bibliography

Bourne, S., and Lewis, E. (1984) Pregnancy after Stillbirth or Neonatal Death. *The Lancet*, July 7: 31–34.

Freud, S. (1917) *Mourning and Melancholia*. Standard Edition, Vol. 14: 243–260.

Hinshelwood, R. D. (1991). *A Dictionary of Kleinian Thought*. London: Free Association Books.

Klein, M. (1929). Personification in the Play of Children. In: The International Psycho-Analytical Library edited by M. Masud Khan No. 103, *Love, Guilt and Reparation and*

Other Works, pp. 199–209. London: The Hogarth Press and the Institute of Psycho-Analysis, 1975.

Klein, M. (1935). A Contribution to the Psychogenesis of Manic-Depressive States. In: The International Psycho-Analytical Library edited by M. Masud Khan No. 103, *Love, Guilt and Reparation and Other Works*, pp. 262–269. London: The Hogarth Press and the Institute of Psycho-Analysis, 1975.

Lewis, E. (1979). Inhibition of Mourning by Pregnancy: Psychopathology and Management. *British Medical Journal*, 7 July, Vol. 2: 27–28.

Papadopoulos, R. (2002). *Therapeutic Care for Refugees: No Place like Home*. London: Karnac Books.

Pozzi, M. (2011). The Use of Observation in Parent-infant Work When Both Parents Have a Diagnosis of Mental Illness. *The International Journal of Infant Observation and Its Application*, Vol. 14(1): 43–60.

Tzŭ, L. (500 BC). *XX. Tao Tệ Ching*. Waley, A., pp. 136–137. London (2010): The Folio Society.

7   Parental mental illness

If you were not here, nothing grows.
I lack clarity. My words
tangle and knot up.
[...]
Look as long as you can at friends you love,
no matter whether that friend is moving away from you
or coming back towards you.

Rumi, circa 1250, p. 52

The literature

Many authors and much research concord with the fact that the external environment including parenting, has a profound effect on the genetic endowment of the infant. "There are three main ways that an infant's health may be damaged: foetal damage, parents' behaviour, and poor physical environment" (Cleaver, 1999, p. 53). "Prenatal adversity and perinatal complications are known to be associated with increased prevalence of child psychiatric disorders" (Hall, 2004 p. 37). "When an infant remains in the care of a mother who is unable to provide adequate care, (s)he may show failure to thrive, often with both developmental delay and retarded growth" (Ibid., p. 37). Mental illness affects parenting capacities: parents cannot be consistent and predictable, emotionally sensitive and able to comfort the distressed infant nor attend to the infant's needs, not to mention the more serious effects of violence, alcohol and drug use on the attachment processes (Ibid., pp. 56–7). Mothers with psychiatric disorders may show anxious, avoidant or disorganised attachment to their infants and be unable to provide understanding and tolerance of their infants needs and developmental changes. However, the protective factor of a secure attachment can be provided by another figure of attachment such as the father or a relative.

Stein (2003) writes: "Although a number of genetic and environmental mechanisms are important in linking parental psychiatric disorder to children's difficulties, there is good evidence that quality of parenting and family interaction are key mediating variables" (p. 243). In an earlier paper, Stein and colleagues

(1998) researched the effect of a psychiatric disorder in the parent, whose thinking process, behaviour and emotionality have been altered, and has lost her or his primary preoccupation for the infant. In particular, parents with eating disorders inevitably affect the infant's intake of food just by being faced with food and having to feed the child. The authors found out that – compared with two control groups – only the children with feeding problems had mothers whose eating habits and attitude to food and to body shape and weight were significantly disturbed. The children who had specific growth problems had mothers with eating disorders.

Crittenden research (1988) linked adult typology with 0-to-24-month-old infant behaviour affirming that maternal and infant behaviour tend to mesh predictably. In particular: controlling/abusive mothers had difficult infants; unresponsive/neglectful mothers had passive infants and inept/marginally maltreating mothers had cooperative infants. The group of cooperative infants behaved in an unpredicted way as some infants were anxious to please, resentful or terrified by their mothers (pp. 142–4).

Rutter et al. conclude that there is little evidence for a major genetic contribution to child psychiatric disorders, apart from early onset major affective disorders, bipolar disorder and anti-social personality disorders. He and his colleagues have explored the "huge diversity of biological consequences – including epigenetic effects" [...] and the "environmental effects on biology" (Rutter et al., 2015, p. 297), in particular the effect on the forming foetus, on its brain growth and birth weight, produced by mothers using alcohol, medications, drugs and smoking, as well as by family stress, traumas, maltreatment etc. There are innumerable neuroscientific studies confirming the effect of the emotional and social environment on the warp and weft of the brain and on the infant's budding personality. To quote the PDM2 (2017): "Appreciating the bidirectional nature of these influences [emotional, social, language, cognitive, regulatory-sensory processing and motor capacities] is crucial to understanding various disorders, tracing their developmental pathways, and making meaningful case formulations and treatment plans" (pp. 625–6).

Paris (2005) writes: "Neither chemical imbalances, psychological adversities, nor a troubled social environment fully account for the development of any mental disorder. Complex interactions between biological, psychological, and social factors are involved in the pathways leading to pathology" (p. 197). Mental disorders arise from the above stressors, continues the author, matched with genetic-temperamental factors leading to vulnerability and family pathology is likely to increase the risk for the development of personality disorders (p. 198). Paris also recognises that the impact of parenting on personality has to be considered in the cultural and societal contexts: family values reflect those of the society and culture the family lives in. He writes that; "abnormal parenting is a risk factor for developing personality disorders. However, [...] the quality of parenting and its impact on the child depends on the larger social environment" (Ibid., pp. 200–1).

Seeman (2004) writes: "The child-rearing environment of the children with mothers with schizophrenia was characterized by less play, fewer learning experiences, less emotional and verbal involvement" (p. 166). Mothers with a diagnosis of schizophrenia and depressive disorders were found to be "less affectively involved with their children than were well mothers" (p. 166).

Norton and Dolan (1996) write that personality-disordered parents may reproduce the negative and deficient parent-child relationship of their own childhood once they become parents themselves (p. 219).

Parents with diagnosis of anti-social personality disorder and borderline personality disorder "are more likely than other parents to exhibit hostile and irritable behaviour towards their children" (Adshead et al., 2004, p. 229).

Steiner (1978) writes that traditionally borderline patients are categorised as being in between psychosis and neurosis: they retain contact with reality, are not formally psychotic but "seem to suffer anxieties of psychotic proportions and to employ primitive mental mechanisms to deal with these" (p. 1).

> The borderline tends to experience the absence of a good object as the presence of a persecution, rather than an experience of loss. He is unable therefore to go through the whole experience of mourning in which, as Freud showed (1917), the self is slowly and painfully detached from the object as the reality of the loss is faced.
>
> (Steiner, 1978, p. 24)

"A failure to use symbols properly leaves the borderline patients without the mental equipment to make reparation and contributes to his hopelessness and despair" (p. 25).

Adshead et al. (2004) found that such parents struggle to relate to their infants and older children in age appropriate ways, mostly due to their difficulty in separating their own needs from those of their offspring. Impulsivity and "ill-considered physical discipline" (p. 229) are used instead of verbal communication and negotiation. These parents – but not all of them – are unable to provide the understanding, continuity and containing function of ordinary parenthood and can be frightening, "dangerous and harmful" (p. 211) to their infants. Parents with these diagnoses reveal to have had abusive childhood themselves suffering with both conduct and hyperactivity disorder.

Tronick (1989) writes that depressed mothers:

> fail to appropriately facilitate their infant's goal-directed activities. Their interactive behaviours and affect are poorly timed or often intrusive. Their affective displays are negative (e.g., anger, sadness, irritability), conveying the message that the infant should change what he or she is doing.
>
> (p. 116)

He continues:

> in abnormal interactions the chronic experience of failure, nonreparation, and negative affect has several detrimental effects on developmental outcome. The infant establishes a self-directed style of regulatory behavior (i.e., turning away, escaping, becoming perceptually unavailable) to control negative affects and its disruptive effects on goal-directed behavior. Indeed, regulation of negative affect becomes the infant's primary goal and preempts other possible goals.
>
> (p. 117)

Jacobsen (2004) writes; "Working with a pregnant psychotic mother can pose specific risks with regard to care of the fetus and future parenting" (p. 114). These mothers can threaten violence towards the unborn infant or suffer from delusional ideas such as a denial of pregnancy. Jacobsen proposes inpatient treatment in the most serious situations or parent-infant psychotherapy, when possible, to help with containing and bonding.

Acquarone (2004) describes several cases of severely mentally ill mothers (puerperal psychosis, schizophrenia, manic breakdown, agoraphobia, borderline, etc.), whose babies had to be looked after by other family members and were subsequently treated in parent-infant psychotherapy as well as medications. The author stresses the importance of observing "the behaviour of the infant, the interrelating (or not) between the infant and the mother, and the quality of his interrelating" (p. 253). Parents "who abuse, start to do so before the baby is born" (p. 254), hence these babies have inborn vulnerabilities and poor constitutional protective factors such as poor capacity to comfort themselves, to self-regulate and to bear frustrations.

The adverse effect of parental mental illnesses on the at-risk baby, who was hyperalert, rigid in her body and showed bonding difficulties, is described in a parent-infant psychotherapy paper by Pozzi (2011).

Maternal depression in infancy, Murray (2009) writes, affects the infant's attachment process, the behaviour as well as its physical, psychological, social and cognitive development. In particular, depressed mothers are impaired or unable to adapt to their baby's needs, to engage and respond to their baby's cues, to baby-talk and mimic in a lively way. These mothers do not offer continuity of emotional care or a safe background of emotional and physical protection.

Mothers with psychiatric disorders tend to have anxious or avoidant children and maltreating parenting leads to disorganised attachment, writes Hall (2004, p. 29).

We read in the PDM2 (2017) that

> Infant attachment "disorganization" refers to an apparent disorganization and confusion when the infant's attachment needs are activated, even though the child is in the caregiver's presence. It has been linked to

frightening or frightened behavior on the part of the parent, so that the infant is trapped in a state that Main (1999) called "fright without solution", in which the parent who should provide a safe haven becomes instead the source of fear.

(p. 510)

The infant is an important agent and with the mother mutually regulates their interaction in a reciprocal dance; we also need to consider the contribution of the genetic disposition of each infant and their temperament, which may contribute or not, to increase risk. As Tronick (1989) writes: "the infant is an agent as well. [...] individual differences in temperament make different infants quite different interactive partners. [...] These sorts of differences place different demands on interactive partners, make infants differentially reactive, and lead to different outcomes" (pp. 117–8). The infant's genetic endowment and temperament, gender, physical attributes, illnesses, emerging personality, resilience etc., can be either an advantage or a disadvantage in the relationship with the ill parent and can contribute to increase the disturbance in the infant or provide protective factors.

"It is often unclear whether an early disorder is best interpreted as an expression of interpersonal relationships or, alternatively, as a potential first sign of individual psychopathology" (Von Klitzing et al., 2015, p. 375).

Neuroscientific studies have made it clear that the quality of early relationships is reflected in the architecture of the brain and thus plays a key role in the development of the child's personality. [...] The younger the child is, the more embedded his or her behavior and biopsychosocial equilibrium are in relationships with parents and other carers. The determination whether any putative manifestation of a mental disorder is truly pathological, or just an expression of normality, can only be made in reference to the child's current stage of development and its characteristic features.

(Ibid.)

Lee and Gotlib (1996) write that

child psychopathology poses a challenge for all family members. The disruption in the child's normal development may interfere with the well-being of all family members, which in turn may lead family members to respond to the disordered child in a negative manner.

(p. 256)

Seneviratne et al. (2004) bring the evidence that childbirth can precipitate bipolar affective or schizoaffective psychosis and while many mothers with mental illnesses can be caring and competent parents, others may be unable to care for their infants, especially when these show "temperamental difficulties" (p. 130), which could be a sign of "inherited mental health problems, which show themselves in subtle ways even during infancy" (Ibid.).

Hall (2004) confirms that

> The child's temperament interacts with the parent's ability to manage him, so that children who are difficult to handle are more likely to develop behaviour problems later in childhood. Babies suffering from narcotic withdrawal syndrome have difficult temperaments and remain very difficult to care for because of irritability, feeding and sleeping difficulties.
>
> (p. 35)

In the following vignettes some of the above concepts are demonstrated.

Clinical vignettes

Philippa, Harold and baby Allister

Philippa and her husband already had a happy and thriving five-year-old son, but Philippa became anxious and depressed during her second pregnancy – which was not planned – and feared not being able to cope with two children. Her worries spanned from emotional to financial and were increased by having received a diagnosis of mental illness in the past. The children's father was present, working and very supportive. Our psychotherapeutic work lasted about six months, starting in the last three months of pregnancy, and it took place in the family home. Mum's presentation, as from my telephone call to arrange a first appointment, was that of an angry and wrongly done woman. She only wanted practical help, that's all she needed, she said. I offered both to liaise with her social worker for practical help and to visit her at home, as she asked me to do. When I arrived, she welcomed me warmly and soon shared all her concerns about her future after the baby's birth i.e. financial, emotional and practical worries. She was of Mediterranean origin, born in Great Britain and had been the victim of much abuse and violence. She was sent to a mental hospital as an adolescent after she had disclosed the abuse and violence received. It was her view that the abuses suffered caused her mental instability and, undoubtedly, this was her true story. However, she had managed to have a healthy family and an impressively wise husband, Harold, whom I had met a few times during my home visits. I offered Philippa a listening and containing space for her accounts, which were at times realistic but puzzling at other times. Her medications made her sleepy and she wanted to stop taking them even before the baby's birth; she felt confused about who her real parents were as she was given different versions from doctors and family members. She would tell me that she used to see ghosts: some were helpful and familiar, others unknown and scary. We agreed that my role would be to help her manage her worries so that the growing baby inside her might be shielded from her excessive anxieties.

She was also keen to learn about mindfulness – which we began to practice together, and it had an immediate, relaxing effect on her. Unfortunately, her baby was due during her parents' long-planned absence and my summer holiday. However, things went well, and the supportive network put in place by her social worker as well as by her husband and his family, gave her a good structure to rely on. Baby Allister was born – as planned – by Caesarean section.

Our work was to be limited in time from the very beginning because I was due to leave the service six months later. This was far from being ideal: Philippa feared that I would not return after the summer holiday and wanted to have my telephone number to call me and to stay in touch with me even after my final departure from the service. We worked a lot on her feelings of abandonment and disappointment with her family and also in relation to me.

Her caring self – which I had already observed when she was interacting with her older son – manifested when Allister was born. She breastfed him competently and bottle-fed him warmly and together with her husband they managed both children quite well.

At that time, I never had any concern about her care and capacity to be available to the baby's demands, neither did her social worker or her health visitor. Philippa related to me as her sounding board to express over and over again her worries, her stories about her past, her anxieties about the future, but she was also able to be in the present with Allister and myself. Mindfulness was a very helpful tool which, to some extent, stopped her wandering mind; she could focus on her breathing, her bodily sensations and once he was born, on Allister resting comfortably in her welcoming lap. He was a "cooperative partner" in this mindfulness practice as he offered her a steady object of observation.

During one home visit, when she was rather anxious and Allister was fretful, we sat and practiced mindfulness together. To her astonishment she did relax, and the baby fell asleep. She said she would go on practicing also in my absence, which she did.

Her ups and downs in moods and her mental worries continued and the great benefits of our time together were hard to sustain when I was not with her.

The time for me to leave approached and she could not envisage letting go of me. She did not want my colleague to take over the work because her depression had gone, she said, and she was happy with her baby. I offered to be available after I left and help her see someone else if needed. It was important that I did not disappear entirely from her life. She was indeed shaken by my premature departure and collapsed due to unpleasant family issues over Christmas time.

Three months later, she telephoned me and I visited her again. She was warm towards me, comfortable with herself and seven-month-old Allister looked a healthy and lively baby. She changed his nappy competently during my visit, then spoon-fed him with home-pureed food. I felt she wanted to show me how well they were doing and spoke of her plan to do an art course at university. She said that mindfulness was helping her when she was anxious and that it calmed her down. She still shared her anxious thoughts about people's gossiping and being unfriendly towards her but her brother – present at that point – encouraged her to ignore such thoughts. Indeed, her mental frailty was there and yet, Allister seemed sheltered at that time. We said goodbye with difficulty, but she did not ask to see me again. Perhaps she was letting go of me at last.

In reflecting on what helped Philippa, I thought it was my quiet reverie, my accepting her imagination and stories, which people were inclined to reject and dismiss as being unreal. I never challenged the truthfulness or not of such statements but linked them in my mind with her early experience of multiple abuses within her family, which she had hurried to recount to me. She felt accepted by me even when she expressed not just her need and love for me, but also negative feelings and criticism of me, followed by intense remorse, concern and apologies. I performed a steady, containing function, which helped her in my presence and shielded Allister to some extent. The time available had, sadly, been too short for her to achieve a more solid trust in herself and less of a belief in her anxious and unreal ideas of being criticised and unloved.

I met them all again when Allister was one year and nine-month-old as I wanted to talk about this writing project. The welcome me warmly and updated me on family life. Philippa was working part-time in evenings and weekend when Harold could look after Allister. Her family relationship had smoothed out and together they were planning a holiday abroad. Allister, a sturdy and well-built toddler took to me immediately, showing me his toys and prancing around excitedly. His parents' loving feelings as well as the healthy boundaries set in place by them were fostering his healthy development and – like his six-year-old brother – seemed lively and well-adapted. Saying goodbye was met with some denial of its emotional impact.

Fiona, Maximillian and baby Bobby

It is difficult to define Fiona's major problem, beyond her diagnosis of personality disorder, and her background of abuse, violence and addiction, which was rather extensive. She wanted to break this cycle and bring up her second baby differently from her first girl, who had been removed from her and brought up by extended family many years earlier. She wanted to give her baby – who was still inside her when the work with us began – a proper home and not the charitable sofa-surfing she had survived on for many years. Our first contact with her happened by phone, she said she was ready to change and be helped by our parent-infant service. The baby's father – also a troubled man – was around and very excited at expecting his first child. With a child psychotherapist colleague, we met Fiona and Max a few times before the planned Caesarean birth and heard about their family histories, concerns and struggles. We also stayed in touch with her by phone, when she could not be driven to the children centre by Max, the baby's father, who always provided her with transport. She had a lot of family support before and after the birth and often stayed at her in-law's or at her twin sister's house.

In the first session with Bobby and Max, she expressed her anxieties about her low moods especially at night but was determined to avoid the post-natal depression (PND) she had suffered from after the birth of her first child. Max poured out all sort of issues, in a non-stop flow, not related to either Fiona or Bobby. Bobby was born by Caesarean and Fiona felt naturally exhausted but pleased and described him affectionately as a "little, greedy, monster, always hungry". He was a particularly endearing baby, who fed well, slept well, hardly ever cried, was always cheerful and smiling; he was surely a constitutionally and genetically healthy and robust baby who, indeed, helped his mother to be good enough for him. Fiona had been heavily medicated before becoming pregnant but stopped taking all her medication during the nine months and valiantly managed the pregnancy well. However, her mood changed after the birth and she was willing to start medications again to prevent a major breakdown with consequences for herself and Bobby. She was also breaking up her partnership with Maxi, whom she had felt intensely furious with, as he was trying to take over the care of their baby and to put her down, thus reminding her of her mother who, Fiona said, had always favoured her twin sister. Therefore, after the first session with Max, she wanted to come alone with Bobby and she would talk a lot about Max and family issues.

Mindfulness had been introduced to them during pregnancy but at this time of intense feelings, it became particularly relevant and useful. We practiced it together when she would become agitated talking about Max, and Bobby too, would reflect on her state by becoming restless and whiney. They both relaxed and calmed down: Fiona felt more at peace and could let go of her intense aversion; Bobby dropped his hyper-vigilance and excessive waving of arms and legs.

The sessions continued and eventually Fiona's annoyance extended to us when, after she missed several sessions, we became concerned and wanted to talk to her health visitor. She broke off contact for several months and when we next saw them again, Bobby was nearly one year old. He looked at us wearily, studied us and looked unsure but as he heard his mum talking freely with us, he ventured to sit on my lap and to play with some toys. Fiona had been able to repair the broken relationship with us and was friendly again. She spoke a lot about her older sister having just died unexpectedly: Fiona's shock, disbelief and regret at not having taken enough of her advice took hold of her. However, she assured us that Bobby was doing well at home, he was feeding and sleeping well.

In sessions we observed Bobby, held in her arms at times, smiling and waving his arms looking happy and well contained by her. He also showed us what a sensitive boy he was, when mum told him not to bang on a glass panel next to the radiator: he looked hurt and bashful.

Complex family issues and dynamics were occurring and Fiona, who had started a specialised group therapy at a local psychiatric hospital, was trying not to be pulled into family problems and separate herself from the family. Bobby was growing healthy and happy and was encouraged to be independent. Fiona was proud of him and felt validated in her new maternal role. They were often at her sister's house, where they talked a lot, fast and non-stop, of anything under the sun, while Bobby enjoyed the company of his young cousins, played and watched television with them.

Relapses occurred in Fiona's life, when disturbing family events gripped her again and she occasionally resumed drinking. We continued our work either at the clinic or at her sister's home – where she was living then – till Bobby was almost two years of age, when my colleague first, then myself after a few months, left the service.

Our departures were experienced with no particular emotions but in a matter-of-fact way: "Oh well, that's life; all things come to an end", Fiona uttered and mentioned all the losses she had to go through since her tender age. She had witnessed her dear father's death, followed by her grandfather's, then friends' death and more recently that of her sister.

In my last home visit, Bobby looked rather sturdy, was sociable with other children and affectionate towards his mother. I felt somewhat reassured that he had been spared a grimmer outcome and that his mother had contained her own disturbance well and managed to protect him enough and help him grow into a robust toddler. On parting Fiona hugged my colleague and later when I also left, she hugged me and thanked us both for the help she received in becoming aware of Bobby and how he could be affected by the environment.

I was only able to talk to Fiona on the phone and not meet her or Bobby personally not because of a lack of trying on my part. She assured me that he was well, thriving and at the moment was staying with his father and grandparents due to her health issues. Fiona was happy about me writing about the work done some years earlier and keen to eventually meet up with me again soon.

Bibliography

Acquarone, S. (2004). *Parent-Infant Psychotherapy: A Handbook*. London: Karnac Books.

Adshead, G., Falkov, A., and Gopfert, M. (2004). Personality Disorder in Parents: Developmental Perspective and Interventions. In: *Parental Psychiatric Disorder*, pp. 217–237, Second edition. Edited by Gopfert, M., Webster, J., and Seeman, M.V., Cambridge: Cambridge University Press.

Cleaver, H., Unell, I., and Aldgate, J. (1999). Child Development and Parenting Capacity. In: *Children's Needs-Parenting Capacity. The Impact of Parental Mental Illness, Problem Alcohol and Drug Use, and Domestic Violence on Children's Development*, pp. 47–98, Edited by Cleaver, H., Unell, I., and Aldgate, J. London: The Stationary Office.

Crittenden, P.M. (1988). Relationship at Risk. In: *The Clinical Implications of Attachment*, pp. 136–174, Edited by Belsky, J. Neswershi, Hillside, NJ: Lawrence Erlbaum Associates, Inc.

Freud, S. (1917). Mourning and Melancholia. *Standard Edition*, Vol. 14: 243–260. The Hogarth Press.

Jacobsen, T. (2004). Mentally Ill Mothers in the Parenting Role: Clinical Management and Treatment. In: *Parental Psychiatric Disorder*, pp. 112–122, C Second |Edition. Edited by Gopfert, M., Webster, J., and Seeman, M.V., Cambridge: Cambridge University Press.

Lee, C.T., and Gotlib, I.H. (1996). Mental Illness and the Family. In: *Handbook of Developmental Family Psychology and Psychopathology*, pp. 243–264, Edited by L'Abate, L., 1994. New York, Chichester, Brisbane, Toronto. Singapore: Wiley & Sons, Inc.

Hall, A. (2004). Parental Psychiatric Disorder and the Developing Child. In: *Parental Psychiatric Disorder*, pp. 22–49, Second edition. Edited by Gopfert, M., Webster, J., and Seeman, M.V., Cambridge: Cambridge University Press.

Main, M. (1999). Epilogue: Attachment Theory: Eighteen Points with Suggestions for Future Studies. In: *Handbook of Attachment: Theory, Research, and Clinical Applications*, pp. 845–888, Cassidy, J. and Shaver, P.R., New York: Guilford Press.

Murray, L. (2009). The Development of Children of Postnatally Depressed Mothers: Evidence from the Cambridge Longitudinal Study. *Psychoanalytic Psychotherapy*, Vol. 23: 185–199.

Norton, K., and Dolan, B. (1996). Personality Disorder and Parenting. In: *Parental Psychiatric Disorder*, pp. 219–232, Edited by Gopfert, M., Webster, J., and Seeman, M.V., Cambridge: Cambridge University Press.

Paris, J. (2005). Parenting and Personality Disorders. In: *Psychopathology and the Family*, pp. 193–204, Edited by Hudson, J.L. and Rapee, R.M., London: Elsevier Ltd.

Psychodynamic Diagnostic Manual, Second Edition PDM-2. (2017) Edited by Lingiardi, V., and McWilliams, N. New York: Guilford Press.

Pozzi, M. (2011). The Use of Observation in Parent-Infant Work When Both Parents Have a Diagnosis of Mental Illness. *The International Journal of Infant Observation and Its Application*, Vol. 14(1): 43–60.

Rumi. (1250 circa). (1995). My Worst Habit. In: *The Essential Rumi*, Translation by Barks, C. with Moyne, J., p. 52. London: Penguin Books.

Rutter, M., and Azis-Clauson, C. (2015). Biology of Environmental Effects. In: *Rutter's Child and Adolescent Psychiatry*, Sixth Edition. pp. 287–301. Oxford: Wiley, J. and Sons, Ltd.

Seeman, M.V. (2004). The Mother with Schizophrenia. In: *Parental Psychiatric Disorder*, pp. 190–200, Edited by Gopfert, M., Webster, J., and Seeman, M.V., Cambridge: Cambridge University Press.

Seneviratne, G., and Conroy, S. (2004). Perinatal Mental Illness: Nature/Nurture. In: *Parental Psychiatric Disorder*, pp. 122–138, Second edition. Edited by Gopfert, M., Webster, J., and Seeman, M.V., Cambridge: Cambridge University Press.

Stein, A., Woolley, H., Challacombe, F., and Feldmann, P. (1998). The Intergenerational Transmission of Disturbance: An Investigation of Mechanisms through the Study of Maternal Eating Disorder. *Infant Observation. The International Journal of Infant Observation and Its Applications*, Vol. 1(3): 31–43.

Stein, A. (2003). The Impact of Parental Psychiatric Disorders on Children. *Editorials, British Medical Journal*, Vol. 327: 242–243.

Steiner, J. (1978). Borderline Personality Disorders. Tavistock Clinic Paper 11. Pamphlet IRN WV.

Tronick, E.Z. (1989). Emotions and Emotional Communication in Infants. *American Psychologist*, Vol. 44(2): 112–119.

Von Klitzing, K., Dohnert, M., Kroll, M., and Grube, M. (2015). Mental Disorders in Early Childhood. Medicine. Continuing Medical Education. *Deutsches Arzteblatt International*, Vol. 112: 375–386.

8 Babies with severe congenital disabilities

Your grief for what you've lost lifts a mirror
up to where you're bravely working.
Expecting the worst, you look, and instead,
here's the joyful face you've been wanting to see.
Your hand opens and closes and opens and closes.
If it were always a fist or always stretched open,
you would be paralyzed.
Your deepest presence is in every small contracting
and expanding,
the two as beautifully balanced and coordinated
as birdwings.

Rumi, circa 1250, p. 174

The literature

Sinason (1993) writes

> When a man and a woman hope for a baby, they hope their baby will be as
> intelligent and fit as they are. [...] For most parents initially, a baby born
> with a disability – especially a mental or multiple one – something has
> gone wrong.
>
> (p. 15)

"Parents need to fantasise and anticipate the future. [...] In such fantasies
very few parents would imagine a child in a wheelchair, a blind child,
a toddler with a profound learning disability" (p. 16), who will grow into disabled adults totally dependent on others. When the baby is born with
a disability, there are often "difficult feelings of shame to deal with between
the marital partners" (p. 28). Sinason continues: "the partners can feel humili-
ated by the fantasy that something damaged or damaging in them has been
passed on. If these feelings are not shared and thought about it can lead to
further stress on the relationship" (p. 28).

What is harder for the baby and the parents is if the shock does not go away. A mother's eyes are the baby's first mirror. [...] Where parents are depressed or feel guilty about the handicap the baby can look up into depressed eyes and take in an image of himself as someone depressing.

(p. 28)

Sinason noticed how common it is for marital relationships to be badly affected to the point of families breaking up. It is more often the father, who disengages himself from the family as being unable to bear the strains of having to care of a handicapped infant and to face what seems to be a failure of his potency (p. 30). Sinason also observed how babies born with physical disabilities may be overprotected for longer than usual and not really encouraged to grow. She describes all sorts of dynamics, which can occur within families: some parents may ignore the disabilities for fear of affecting the chance of the infant's potential development; others blame the healthy child for not making extra allowances for the disabled infant; others tend to ignore the healthy siblings to devote more time and energy to the sick infant.

Emanuel (1997) writes about the primary disappointment of a mother who, instead of having a beautiful baby – the baby she had phantasised and hoped to have had – she is instead faced with a disabled baby. Severe difficulties in their relationship are likely to be established and to endure in the child's life. Some of these dynamics and issues were embedded in the family here described.

Clinical vignette

Felicity and twin-babies Davina and Christiana

Felicity found it hard to start the work with me – despite expressing an interest – and would forget, cancel or double-book her appointments. Born in an African country, she had been raised by a loving grandmother, having had her mother abandon her as a baby. She was sent to Europe at the age of nine when her grandmother became ill and then died. In Europe she had unsatisfactory, fostering experiences with extended family and with other adults, till she moved away to live alone: she was about 17 then.

When she was referred to our Parent-Infant Service, she had just given birth to twins – one with a congenital syndrome – and was afraid of not bonding with them as well as of repeating her family history of maternal rejection, neglect and abandonment. She came to our service when the twins were two-months old, having already had some short-term counselling over the issue of bonding but needing more in-depth work. The babies' father had taken hardly any interest in them to begin with, so Felicity cut him off completely from seeing them, feeling ill-treated just like she had felt with her own father, whom she had only met once or twice in her earliest life. She revealed this in the course of our brief work.

In our first session, she placed the twins on the floor mat where we were sitting and gave a bottle to Davina – the sick baby – to feed herself, while she held and fed Christiana in her arms. In an incongruous way, she said that she was aware of giving the sick twin more time and attention as the baby needed it and of leaving Christiana to her own devices. On this occasion, she let baby Davina struggle to hold the bottle with her fingers of her deformed fist stuck together. It was part of Davina's rare, congenital syndrome to have fingers joint together in a fist and a face larger than normal and somewhat deformed.

She was awaiting surgery to have her fingers separated. Christiana smiled a lot and gurgled happily. I said to baby Davina how hard it was to struggle to hold the bottle and that she must have felt very alone on that cushion. As I observed her, I wondered to myself if the mother was already projecting her own experience of loneliness and abandonment onto her less-fortunate baby, as well as onto myself, earlier in our hit-and-miss meetings at the children centre, when it took such a long time to come to our Clinical Service and engage with me. She opened up to me and cried in remembering her good grandmother, who was now dead and greatly missed, but whose loving care was kept alive inside her. She was able to rely more on that good, early experience and to let go of her anger and resentment at her other neglectful and emotionally abusive experiences. In this first session I introduced mindfulness, which Felicity was interested in learning and we practiced it together in sessions. It gave her the experience of observing her own body sensations and both her babies' response to her calmer state: they looked at her while being very still and with enquiring expressions. She also joined a mindfulness group for mothers and babies.

We met only four more times, which were spread out over the following eight months; this was due to her forgetting sessions, cancelling or not attending due to Davina's appointments at the children's hospital. However, her pattern of cancelling, not attending or double-booking sessions lessened once she knew we had a limited period of time available as I was leaving the service nine months from the beginning of our work. From our second meeting, she seemed to have dried out after that initial, emotional encounter and had hardly anything to recount about their week or to explore with me. After Davina's hand operation, Felicity reported that everything was fine. In our third session, she placed the babies against a cushion on the floor next to us. Christiana was very chatty and chirped away and Davina copied her. Then Christiana pulled Davina's sleeve up but her mother told her not to. I wondered silently whether Christiana was trying to involve Davina in some movement and perhaps looking at her operated-on hands, while the mother was talking about it. Davina, who was more physically impaired than her twin, was very present to the happenings in her surroundings: she looked at her sister pulling up her sleeve or moved her head in the direction of her mother's voice, when her name was been called out.

We spoke of the importance for babies to know their fathers and this was enough for Davina to contact the babies' paternal grandmother, who spoke to her son i.e. the babies' father. He started to show more interest in them and offer a small, supportive financial sum to the mother. Perhaps our sessions had unblocked something in Felicity, who could make peace internally with the girls' father. In the session she grew able to share her attention and involvement with both twins more equally – perhaps in identification with me. Yet, she still said she needed to give more time and attention to the sick baby. There, on the mat, Davina was more still, as being unable to move but she was rather vociferous, while Christiana more adventurous, mobile and keen to engage her sister. Felicity revisited her young years in Africa again and again sadly, and idealised her life there, which she felt to have been so much better probably because of her grandmother's good care and love for her. I think it was that loving care that equipped her with inner strength and capacity to look after her twins and their unusual problems. In fact, she recognised that she was a good parent to her babies and managed her life competently.

She developed a rather robust relationship with them both, which included a good dose of teasing. This, at times, concealed frustration and annoyance and we were able to address it and to reduce a potentially unhealthy attitude. She was very interested in hearing about babies self-regulating and – for example – turning away when stimulations become too intense: she would no longer perceive that as a rejection.

Felicity was keen to return to work when the twins were about nine months old. Sadly, I could not influence the timing of such a separation, despite alerting her on how crucial a time that was in babies' development. Her need to return to work then, surmounted anything else. She had planned and found suitable childminding for her babies and was very pleased that "she had given them a good mother" – i.e. herself – and managed to be different from her own mother. Her old experience of maternal rejection was told and re-told and re-lived, indeed, again, when I had to leave the service. It was nine months after we began our work and she was nine years when she had to leave her beloved grandmother and her country: what an amazing and painful coincidence! It gave us the chance to work more on separation, loss, abandonment and rejection, all very deeply felt issues for Davina. It was also possible for her to just feel some annoyance, too, at my leaving, and not just excruciating sadness. However, she made me leave before my actual leaving day – interestingly she thought I was leaving two weeks earlier than I was due – she was somehow getting rid of me before I was due to leave the service. Perhaps this was her way of taking control of a painful situation and making me feel like the discarded one, a too well-known, emotional experience for her.

She assured me that she would remember what we had done together, just like she had carried her grandmother's loving care inside her.

I met them again on the occasion of writing this book as I wanted her to read, comment and approve of what I had written. It was rather laborious to arrange this due to misunderstandings about dates and cancellations, similar to our earlier encounters. Eventually, we met at their home on a sunny say. Felicity welcomed me warmly and was very happy to see me again. The twins aged two-and-four months were sitting in their high chairs, munching away at their chicken nuggets and chips, glued to a cartoon television programme and ignoring us both. They remained there till the end of their lunch, when the mother set them free to roam around their large bedsitter. Eventually they acknowledged me and played with me and we looked at books together, while Felicity updated me on their progress.

Everything was moving along steadily: the girls were well settled with the same childminder two or three days a week, depending on Felicity's work; Davina was still undergoing operations on her head and hands at the local children's hospital; Felicity had stopped their unreliable father from seeing the twins, who only wanted to visit them when it suited him and with no consideration for the children's needs. Felicity had good plans for herself to train and work with children with disabilities "I have all this experience with Davina", she said and indeed, she had been managing to bring up the twins valiantly through difficulties and loneliness: she had been a very dedicated mother indeed! She felt valued by being part of a book and spoke to the twins about it with pride and self-recognition: she was looking forward to celebrating its publication. We parted with some hesitation and sadness stayed with me for some time after.

Bibliography

Emanuel, L. (1997). Facing the Damage Together. *Journal of Child Psychotherapy*, Vol. 23(2): 279–302.

Rumi. (circa 1250). *Birdwings. The Essential Rumi*. Translated by Coleman Barks with John Moyne (1995), p. 174. London: Penguin Books.

Sinason, V. (1993) Pregnancy and Fear of Disability. In: Tavistock Clinic Series Editor: Elsie Osborne *Understanding Your Handicapped Child*, pp. 15, 16, 28, 30. Rosendale Press: London.

9   Fathers

It is a wise father that knows his own child
Shakespeare, *The Merchant of Venice*, 2ii

A literature review

"'What are fathers for? To be the other parent' said psychiatrist Sebastian Krea-mer" (Daws and de Rementeria, 2015, p. 78).

The presence of fathers in infant-parent psychotherapy has become a topic of interest in recent years: he can be present physically or virtually, in the mother's mind, and this creates the much-needed triangular space where the infant can develop. Having said that, it is now well recognised that both parents can perform the maternal function of being tender and receptive and the paternal one, of being firm and structuring. Both parents can alternate in these essential ways of being, as growing up requires that the baby accept the presence and care from the mother and father, or a third person. The baby internalises the way parents relate and function as a couple, not just as separate individuals. One of the therapist's roles is to embody both maternal and paternal functions of intuitive reverie and acceptance as well as of bringing words, symbols, playfulness and structure into the primary dyad. Here follows a detailed and updated literature review on the topic of fathers followed by clinical vignettes showing both the importance and value of the paternal, physical presence for the psychic survival of the mother-baby dyad and the devastating effect of the absent and/or rejecting father.

Many psychoanalytic authors, going back to Freud and Klein, contribute to this topic starting with the infantile origin of the interest in the father: his role and functions, absence and loss, abusive and malevolent presence. The infant may either identify with an external, father figure, who acts as a protector against an engulfing relationship with the mother; or internalise a paternal function, which allows the infant to have a relationship with his father in the mind; or desire the actual father instead of the excessively anxiety-provoking mother, and this may lead to some difficulties in developing a secure sexual identity.

Acquarone (2004) in her book *Infant-Parent Psychotherapy*, thinks that the mother's mind offers a triangular space to the infant by having resolved her Oedipal conflict and holding her own mother and father as a couple in her mind. This allows the infant to have space in his growing mind for his father to exist – whether father is physically present or not. The quality of the parental relationship and of the father are perceived through the mother's mind. "Paternal reverie" (p. 42) creates an attention to both mother and baby and allows the father to revisit his past as well as imagine the future. She also writes about abusive fathers, who are unable to have a "paternal reverie", due to their problematic or pathological upbringing, but can actually abuse the baby's mother as well as the baby during pregnancy and after birth.

Baradon and his colleagues at the Anna Freud Centre in their books *The Practice of Psycho-analytic Parent-Infant Psychotherapy* (2005), and *Working with Fathers in Psychoanalytic Parent-Infant Psychotherapy* (2019) report their clinical, psychoanalytic parent-infant work and that of their many colleagues, regarding the value of the father's presence and, occasionally, also of the necessity of his absence. As well as the many roles of fathers in the baby's life, they write about absent fathers, who can still be kept alive for the baby by the mother. Good, caring images of fathers or malign, abusive ones are transmitted by mothers in a more or less conscious manner to the small child, who will internalise and believe such maternal representations of the father.

Barrows (2004) in his paper "Fathers and Families: Locating the Ghost in the Nursery", explores the father's ghosts in the nursery as well as the fundamental role of the couple relationship and its quality, which becomes internalised by the infant. The parent–child dyads are to be addressed in the treatment but also broadened to the relationship the parents have. Barrows presents several clinical vignettes and explores the difficulties presented by parents in protecting the parental couple and tolerating excluding the infant. Different infants and small children have their own specific individuality, characteristics and different attachment patterns to their mother and father, which all contribute differently to family dynamics.

Brazelton and Cramer (1991) in their book *The Earliest Relationship*, describe the attachment process to the baby in fathers-to-be, and this is – just as it is for the mother – influenced by the father's childhood experiences. Learning to be a father is a developmental process, which produces many feelings that need to be tolerated. The father's potency is expressed when conception occurs and a sense of shock as well as pleasure may derive from this new state. Also, there can be feelings of exclusion during pregnancy, envy for the woman's capacity to grow and bear a baby in her womb; a different sense of responsibility vis-à-vis the partner and the new-born; competitiveness in either the care of the baby or in getting the partner's attention; acceptance of the different involvement and type of relationship with the baby than the mother's. The authors affirm that the baby has different attachments to the father and the mother. Support of the mother-infant dyad as well as buffering against the intrusions from the outer world are often expected of a new father.

Cowan and Cowan (2001) in their paper "A Couple Perspective on the Transmission of Attachment Patterns", research the quality of the couple functioning on the young child's capacity to adapt to social situations. The father's role and the fit between the two attachment histories of the parents affect the child's emotional development and adaptation. The couple relationship and their parenting ways are correlated and the improvement of the former leads to an improvement of the latter.

Daws and de Rementeria (2015) in their book *Finding Your Way with Your Baby*, dedicate a whole chapter to fathers: the process of becoming a father, of offering a third position, and a "particular relationship to the baby and to the mother-and-baby couple" (p. 78). "It is not just a cliché that mothers hold babies protectively in their arms, while fathers are the ones to throw the baby up in the air, to offer challenging, exciting play that includes mastery over fear" (p. 86). "A tactful father can make mother and baby feel that he can look after them both without undermining an exhausted mother's authority" (p. 87). However, the father's new role as a protector and provider, may also stir up the equally disquieting memories and emotions from his childhood and the biochemical changes that the father, too, undergoes, when living close to his pregnant partner and caring for the baby after the birth. Fathers, the authors continue, have the same physiological response to the baby's crying as mothers do and show the same sensitivity to feeding the baby as mothers. Research show that there are hormonal changes in men too, "Prolactin increases feelings of protectiveness and concern and this goes up in men who are living with their partners during pregnancy. Their testosterone also goes down after birth, which is likely to reduce sex drive" (Ibid., p. 43).

Emanuel and Bradley (2008) in their book *What Can the Matter Be?* remind the reader that the maternal function is that of being more receptive while the paternal role is that of structuring and transforming what is received, of setting limits and being firm. Mothers and fathers can embody both functions in the absence of either of them. An absent father can be powerfully present in the mother's mind either as a benign or a malign presence. The child too can be well aware of the father's absence and often takes his place by positioning himself in bed next to Mum. The Oedipal triangulation is, thus, skewed and the child is deprived of the possibility of internalising a united and creative, parental couple.

Fivaz-Depeursinge and Corboz-Warnery (1999) in their book *The Primary Triangle*, observe the infant's – as young as three and four months – capacity for triangulation i.e. for engaging with both parents simultaneously, making what they call "triangular bids". In the LTP (Lausanne Trilogue Play) parents are asked to play and interact with their babies in a semi-structured situation of being seated together in the same room. The micro-analysis of the video shows that the three-person communication between the infant and the parents can take place very early on.

Gerhardt (2004) in her book *Why Love Matters*, writes mostly about mothers but also refers to the effect of the quality of the relationship between parents and child on the structure and biochemistry of the baby's brain: the parents' behaviour will be encoded on the baby's neural pathways and the baby will relate according to such a now-physically-engrained relationship. The baby's brain also encodes the parental relationship as well as the parents' separate relationship with the baby.

Kraemer (2005) in the chapter Narratives of Fathers and Sons: "There is No Such Thing as a Father", emphasises the idea that the many qualities traditionally belonging to one sex or the other, can be shared in a way that varies from couple to couple and from time to time even in the same couple. The father's participation liberates the mother and also has a direct effect on his perception of himself as a real man and the infant experiences being looked after, wanted and being loved by both parents.

Lieberman et al. (2015) in their book *Don't Hit My Mommy!*, trace the origin of an aggressive stance

> to the earliest years of childhood, to experiences of helplessness and pain that instil in the child a conviction that being on the offensive is the best defence. Witnessing violence and being the victim of violence shatter the child's confidence that his well-being matters and that adults will take care of him. [...] Millions of children who are exposed to family violence share Sandra's internal dilemma of yearning for safety while simultaneously learning that the people she loves make each other cry.
>
> (p. 1)

Although the authors are very careful in not writing about violent fathers directly and are more general in mentioning family violence, the title of this book speaks for itself.

McHale (2007) in *When Infants Grow Up in Multiperson Relationship Systems*, is keen to observe co-parenting and family alliance patterns, as he calls them, such as "patterns of competitiveness, verbal sparring and active interference amongst the components" (p. 374). He describes different family types with the child at the centre, and parents who vary from positive co-parenting in a co-operative connection with each other, to parents who only engage with the infant, but not with each other, or have very different levels of engagement with the infant or may be disengaged from the infant. Marital distress is reflected in parenting issues: adequate dyadic parental engagement may not be adequate enough when it comes to the whole family set up i.e. to the triangular context.

Perelberg in her erudite book *Murdered Father, Dead Father* refers to the work by Freud, Lacan and others on the passage from the narcissistic father who possessed women by terror and was murdered by their sons, and the dead father, i.e. the internalised father, who prohibits the son from seducing and possessing mother and sisters, thus establishing law and culture. The Oedipal constellation with the introduction of the "third" (father or any "others", including mother herself), interrupts and contains the engulfing and erotic feelings in the mother-infant dyad so that the infant's intense and exclusive desire for the mother is contained and transformed.

Pozzi (2003) in her book *Psychic Hooks and Bolts*, presents vignettes where fathers have different positions. We read about an authoritarian father in conflict with a permissive wife, who indulges Rosy with her bowel and soiling problem or a father able to break the enmeshed relationship between the mother and a three-year-old boy, indulged by her and in his feminine identification due to uncontained separation anxieties. The father's claiming more of the child for himself provided the mother with the separateness and robustness that allowed Ron to develop along a heterosexual trajectory. A supportive and healthier father helps the mentally ill mother manage the baby with ordinary, daily tasks and provides a more secure attachment to Bonny when the mother is admitted to hospital.

Raphael-Leff (2003) in her book *Parent-Infant Psychodynamics*, refers to the crucial need for mothers to have emotional and practical support from a partner and the degree and quality of involvement she has from such a partner. A partner, who is envious of either the mother's capacity to give birth and nurture, or of her relationship with the infant, or who withdraws to protect his/her own boundaries, increases the burden and pressure on the new mum. A scenario can also appear where the partner's possessiveness, sexual demands and violence can take over family life. The main carer is exposed to a dangerous situation of being entrapped in a dyadic relationship where the baby, too, may become invested with dangerous projections by his unsupported mother.

Paul and Thomson Salo (2014) in their book *The Baby as Subject*, bring our attention to fathers who abuse their babies causing them huge damage especially in the absence of a protective mother. They mention the interplay of maternal traumatic childhood experience with maternal projections on the baby in the present, which requires early psychotherapeutic intervention to undo the intergenerational repetition of trauma and abuse.

Vallino (2004) in her book *Essere Neonati* (*To Be Infants*, title translated by Pozzi) focuses on the father's role in helping to mediate and modulate possible impasses between mother and baby. Growing up requires not only a capacity to manage separation but also the acceptance of an alternating relationship with the mother and with non-maternal figures, who offer different things to the baby. The father can be a playmate and bring the ludic function as well as experimenting and showing the baby new things, thus offering another attachment figure to the infant.

Von Klitzing et al. (1999) in their paper "The Role of the Father in Early Family Interaction," study the co-parenting relationship before the baby's birth, i.e. the triangular capacities in young parents to imagine their future as a family with three people. The parents' subjective views about their parenthood and the unborn child are systematically analysed during pregnancy, focusing on the importance of fathers for the development of the infant and the family as anticipated in the parental fantasies. These representational dimensions are compared with the quality of dyadic and triadic parent–child interactions observed after the child is born. A specific and significant correlation is found between aspects of the father's representational world and the four-month-old infant's capacity to get into a well-balanced contact with both parents in a triadic interactional setting.

Clinical vignettes

Harriette, Frank and baby Henry

Henry aged five-and-a-half months, was referred by his GP because his mother Harriette, was unsure about their bonding, felt surreal in having a baby and almost depersonalised. Her post-natal depression was serious and worrying all the professionals around her. She had lost her competence as a professional worker and carer of babies and young children and could not recognise herself as a mother. Henry was left in his cot, only picked up or stimulated by his father and paternal grandmother, whom Harriette and baby Frank were living with. She allowed her partner, Henry's father, to help her a great deal with Henry, while she sadly perceived her mother-in-law's help as a further sign of her inadequacy and failure as a mother. She revealed that she felt she was still an adolescent, very close to her father and could not be a proper mother to a baby. How could she do that? Her own parents were also involved and caring when she visited them occasionally, but they lived in another far-away town. Harriette would have preferred to live with them but felt that Henry needed his own father close by.

Her presentation in the first session at a local Children Centre, was alarming: she was hunched over, had no eye contact with me or with Harry, she was cut off and not responding to him crying. She was very thin and anxious; her sentences were fragmented and words chopped in half. She was ridden with doubts, self-reproach and guilt: "Was it the right thing to have kept the pregnancy?" she wondered and concluded that she was not capable of being a mother, she was not bonding and felt nothing for her baby; she was worried that she "was already damaging his brain and general development". There was no obvious risk of her wanting to hurt or kill herself or her baby – a well-known fact in severely post-natally depressed mothers – but a possibility I nevertheless explored thoroughly with her.

In the session, the baby was plonked on the mat and there he stayed still for some moments; eventually he moved vigorously to reach out for her but she was cut off from his attempts to reach out so he turned himself round to where my voice was coming from, looked at, and reached out for me. I said: "You're looking at your Mum and reaching out for her, but she is too worried and cannot play with you!" I then addressed Harriette: "He knows you are "adultese" for her. When she spoke to him, it was as if she spoke to a stranger and not to her baby, who was lying there on the mat and reaching out for another human being.

Their story enfolded: he was born suddenly in the taxi that was taking them to the local hospital. This proved to be a real shock to Harriette who, as she said, had no time to prepare for his delivery: he just came out so unexpectedly and fast! She did not encourage her mother, who was busy with her other ill son in hospital, to be with her, when she was sick with stomach pains in the special care unit. I said that as well as feeling low, incapable, bewildered and unprepared to have this baby, she also felt that she was unable to be a mother and a failure: all this prevented her from just giving herself a chance.

A freeing factor in this very first session was both noticing Harriette's hidden, intense resentment towards this baby and putting it into words to them both: "Mum is annoyed with you at times because Mum is very tired and doesn't understand that you want her to pick you up and cuddle you!" After an initial surprise, she was able to access her angry feelings, no longer projected onto me, and to admit to them. Almost magically, her good feelings towards him were somewhat freed and she looked at Henry, gave him a rattle and engaged with him a little more.

A further comment which struck home, was about her identification with a lonely baby-self left in an intensive care unit in hospital with no mother around. At this point, she picked up wiggly and agitated Henry, sat him on her knees and he could relax to some extent. This could have been a proof of her importance to him, but instead she insisted that she was not a good mother.

Together we also practiced mindfulness, which I explained and demonstrated to her. We both observed our bodies and felt our sensations as we breathed in and out slowly and calmly, while at the same time observing Henry with a less entangled eye. He quite soon gave up his restlessness completely and settled in his mother's lap, turning towards her face.

At home – and when he was rarely free to come to the centre – her partner Frank continued to be a very helpful presence: he supported her practically even though it was hard for him to understand both the depth of her disturbance, which had required a specialist intervention of parent-infant psychotherapy, and to believe that it would get better.

During my home visits, I had a chance to meet her extended family and could understand Harriette's feelings that their earlier help had turned into taking over her maternal care, as if she still needed it and that she was not recognised as a capable mother. Through ups and downs in her self-esteem, Harriette preserved and improved her emotional availability to Henry and was determined "to get stronger", she said, and not get caught up in painful family tensions and generational differences.

Henry grew into a sturdy boy, at times "too much on the go", which together we were able to rectify and contain. He was a healthy, curious, inquisitive, sociable boy, who muttered sounds and half words and by the age of two was settled well in nursery. It was very heartening when, during a home visit, I observed his parents changing his nappy in a loving and cooperative way, helping each other and with neither competition nor reciprocal putting down.

Harriette's positive and movingly idealised transference towards me and her steady commitment contributed, together with other helping hands, to contain her quasi-psychotic anxieties and fears and she learnt to enjoy and love her baby. His sturdy constitution and good character contributed to the resolution of her earlier post-natal depression and helped her to become a fully-fledged, competent and proud mother.

I had the good fortune to meet Harry and Harriette again when he was four-and-a-half years old, on the occasion of writing this piece, which I wanted mum and dad to read. We met at a coffee shop and had lunch together. Harry looked at me shyly, to begin with, but soon we made friends and he spoke freely and enjoyed his sausage roll and drink with us. He was healthy, sturdy, happy and well settled in his home life with Mum, his maternal grandparents and seeing his father together with Mum on most weekends. After being initially upset, he also settled in well in the local nursery, where Mum also worked a few hours. He was described by Mum as being very affectionate and concerned if someone was hurt, upset, in pain; but he was also able to protest vociferously, as I was witness to, when he could not get his own way. The warm relationship between him and his mother was nourishing for them both and Mum, on reading my piece, wished she had not been so unwell when he was a baby; she said he had done her good and helped her to be more open and sociable with people around her. She loved him and rejoiced in his presence thoroughly.

Donna, Abe and baby Thomas

It was hard to engage Donna and the initial appointments were cancelled. When we finally met with a colleague of mine, Donna was pregnant with her fifth child and was unsure whether she wanted to keep the pregnancy. This child's father, like the other children's fathers, was absent from her life and she, herself, had never met her own father but was not bothered about it, she assured us. All her other children, born when she was very young, were going through deep difficulties with drugs, mental illnesses and homelessness.

She was referred to our infant-mental health service when her short Cognitive Behavioural Therapy (CBT) treatment was coming to an end, but more work was needed in view of Donna's recent pregnancy and ongoing depression.

The beginning of our work was nearly aborted as we managed to upset her by enquiring about fathers and their absence too much. However, she managed to come back and the work continued. Donna's impenetrable look, her emotional disconnection, the manic outbursts of giggling, were noticeable as well as the pervasive feeling that she was in a vacuum and, deep down, unsure of her identity. However, once she engaged with us, she attended with ups and downs and opened up more freely: having decided that she could not go through an abortion, she came to accept that she wanted to try and be different with this baby. She had been too permissive with her other children and her partners, and this had led her to always being alone.

Being aware of her difficulties with intimate relationships, she worried about her attachment to her baby-in-the-womb and her ambivalent feelings. Gradually she was able to get in touch with her sadness at her baby's father having rejected her when she became pregnant and she went through the delivery more peacefully.

She had been tearful for a few weeks after giving birth to Thomas and she put it down to her hormones, but for several sessions, she would come alone and speak unkindly and not affectionately about the baby, which may have pointed towards post-natal depression. Feeling rejected and unwanted were deep wounds for Donna and we had to help her not to pass onto her baby her own feelings of rejection, while we had to endure her comings and not coming with patience and resilience.

Eventually she brought the baby to our sessions and we noticed that she was not able to look into his eyes, but glided away, looking depressed and he was turning away from her face. She revealed that looking at him reminded her of his abandoning father. Yet she felt no anger towards him, just sad that Thomas would have no father; she rationalised and accepted his father's decision not to be involved with one more child in his life.

For many sessions, Thomas looked very still, frozen, uninvolved and avoided visual contact with his Mum's face. When she felt instinctively drawn to him, we noticed that she would push away from a closer contact because she "did not want to disturb him", she said, when we verbalised this observation. Apparently, even at home, he never looked at her. We tried to explore what he might be seeing in her eyes that was disturbing, hence his gaze-avoidance. Donna shrugged her shoulders and had no thoughts or imagination.

My colleague and I carried her projection that one of us was "the soother" and the other one "the challenger", so she described us. With some effort, though, she was indeed able, on one occasion, to have a whole session with only the challenger and to survive it well!

Thomas was still reported to be sleeping a lot and spending much time with his maternal grandmother or with Donna's older daughter. Our anxiety that Thomas might develop autistic-like defences was shared with Donna and we decided to be rather active and educational in our approach, as well as making descriptive comments about the relational dynamics going on between her and her baby. We suggested that she engaged him in playful, baby-like exchanges with hands, rattles, soft toys etc. and looked into his face and eyes smilingly and happily, perhaps visualising a flower or something nice, not memories of Thomas's abandoning fathers. We also introduced mindfulness of breathing exercises to encourage her to look at him and observed him in a neutral and benevolent way, while breathing in and out slowly.

We became reassured when we noticed that Thomas was selectively avoiding his mother's face but could look at us fully and intently. Donna began – out of her own initiative – to sing lovely lullabies, when he was restless and sleepless: he had, in fact, moved out of a still and depressed state and become hypervigilant and agitated. But he was still not looking at her! She gradually came to terms with trying to involve the rejecting father and sent him photos and videos of Thomas, but for a long time there was no response by him to her hard-won initiative. Although this was another painful experience of rejection for Donna, at least she said she could put her mind to rest and give up on any hope to involve the father.

Thomas was nine months old, when Donna had let go of any feelings, hopes and wishes regarding his father and could look at Thomas as a little boy in his own right, no longer a reminder of a rejecting father and partner. She made herself look at him in the eyes but he was still zooming out and rejecting her but she affirmed that she was not feeling rejected by him! She told us that that he was probably picking up on her sadness, which had to do mainly with the thought that he would never meet his father. We gave her permission to feel and express her sad feelings as this awareness was already a healing factor: she then bounced Thomas on her legs then held him firmly in her arms and, while humming a tune, he fell asleep there. Her depression improved through ups and downs, sessions not attended or forgotten, and eventually she grew sincere affection towards Thomas and curiosity about his emotional development.

A turning point occurred when Donna spoke at length about her most troublesome daughter – Thomas being thirteen months old then – who never stopped blaming her for all the mistakes she had made with her. Donna had to go through a grieving process as she felt a bad, inadequate mother, then full of sadness, regret, guilt and a self-reflective sense of responsibility vis-à-vis her daughter. This new state of mind propelled her to work even harder at her relationship with Thomas; she changed and became deeply concerned and a reparatory-type guilt motivated her to engage more with Thomas, play with him, set appropriate limits and hold him when he was hyperactive and uncontained. He would now go to her for comfort and cuddles, something new for him, and they became able to look at each other's eyes for some moments. We still noticed that Thomas's' eyes became fixed and frozen-like at times. Her eyes had also been affected by an eye illness and could not focus ordinarily, which did not help.

In the course of our psychotherapy, Donna had to undergo a number of eye interventions and, all in all, things slowly improved and they eventually could look at each other properly. She would face me and my colleague directly into our eyes and reported good progress with Thomas. In sessions she played, stopped him when he chucked toys around and disciplined him firmly and warmly. She eventually, decided with deep trepidation, to contact Thomas's father Abe again, as "life was too short" to hold onto grudges. We worked on the possibility that he may not respond again and whether she would manage that further rejection. However, he did reply and plans to meet were made: he, too was ready to meet this young son of his and to become involved constructively in his life. They met and Thomas took to him and they played for a few hours with mother being present. She began to trust Abe more and could let Thomas spend a night there after they got to know each other better.

Our work was coming to a natural end as things had improved on all fronts, Thomas was approaching his second year and Donna contemplated resuming an old friendship, which was to become an intimate and nourishing relationship with a loving man. This was a sign of her internal, real progress as dating this old, dear friend who had been around her at her most difficult times, testified that she had internalised a benign paternal figure and she could risk getting emotionally involved again.

To conclude, coming to her session had been hard indeed, and Donna had openly admitted to often feeling reluctant, but being determined to make things better: "then it helps and I feel happier for having come", she had admitted bravely and honestly. We provided the emotional and containing backdrop which she had never experienced in her life and having this fifth child assisted by the parent-infant psychotherapy gave her a new opportunity to repair much about her past as a child, a mother and a partner. The therapeutic work brought the father or paternal function of giving structure and symbolism back into the mother-infant dyad. This occurred by talking about absent father figures, by bearing without retaliating her rejections expressed by not attending and dis-appearing for sessions, and by us performing as well as a maternal, containing function, also the paternal, composite functions of providing a third position, boundaries, challenges and separateness.

I met Donna and Thomas again – this time in their home – and for the pur-pose of sharing what I had written about our psychotherapeutic work done in the past. Thomas presented as a bright, alert and exuberant child, running around on his scooter both indoors and out in the street. He spoke well and responded to his mother's request fairly appropriately. He was rather unpleasant towards me when I first arrived and we put it down to him not-knowing me but also to not wanting to share his mother: he paused only fleeting next to me to look at a book that I was trying to read to him. Donna only reprimanded him about his rudeness but did not stop him running around on his scooter. She was still struggling with ups and downs due to family preoccupation and a recent and mysterious cot-death of a baby in her family. Walking in the streets and Thomas pedalling his scooter freely proved helpful and relaxing for us all. Donna's was planning to do a brief training which will allow her to patrol schools, streets and public places. She was grateful about our meeting and hoped to stay in touch.

Bibliography

Acquarone, S. (2004). *Infant-Parent Psychotherapy.* London and New York: Karnac Books.

Baradon, T. (Editor) (2019a). *Fathers.* London and New York: Routledge.

Baradon, T. (Editor) (2019b). *Working with Fathers in Psychoanalytic Parent-Infant Psychotherapy.* Oxon and New York: Routledge.

Baradon, T., with Biseo, M. (2016). Fathers. In: *The Practice of Psycho-analytic Parent-Infant Psychotherapy*, pp. 109–114. London and New York: Routledge.

Baradon, T., with Broughton, C., Gibbs, I., James, J., Joyce A. and Woodhead, J. (2005). *The Practice of Psycho-analytic Parent-Infant Psychotherapy*. Hove and New York: Routledge.

Barrows, P. (2004). Fathers and Families: Locating the Ghost in the Nursery. *Infant Mental Health Journal*, Vol. 25(5): 408–423.

Brazelton, T.B., and Cramer, B.G. (1991). *The Earliest Relationship*. London: Karnac Books.

Cowan, P., and Cowan, C. (2001). A Couple Perspective on the Transmission of Attachment Patterns. In: *Adult Attachment and Couple Psychotherapy*, pp. 62–82. Edited by Clulow, C., London: Brunner-Routledge.

Daws, D., and de Rementeria, A. (Editors) (2015). Figuring Out Fatherhood. In: *Finding Your Way with Your Baby*, pp. 78–91. Hove and New York: Routledge.

Emanuel, L., and Bradley, E. (2008). *What Can the Matter Be?* London: Karnac Books.

Fivaz-Depeursinge, E., and Corboz-Warnery, A. (1999). *The Primary Triangle*. New York: Basic Books.

Gerhardt, S. (2004). *Why Love Matters*. London and New York: Routledge.

Kraemer, S. (2005). Narratives of Fathers and Sons: "There Is No Such Thing as a Father". In: *Narrative Therapies with Children and Their Families: A Practitioners Concepts and Approaches*, pp. 115–132. Edited by Vetere, A. and Dowling, E. London and New York: Brunner-Routledge.

Lieberman, A.F., Ghosh Ippen, C., and Van Horn, P. (Editors) (2015). Introduction. In: *Don't Hit My Mommy!*, pp. 1–5. Washington, DC: ZERO to THREE.

McHale, J. (2007). When Infants Grow Up in Multiperson Relationship Systems. *Infant Mental Health Journal*, Vol. 28(4): 370–392.

Paul, C., and Thomson Salo, F. (2014). Sara: Psychotherapy with a Mother-infant Dyad with a Background of Violence. In: *The Baby as Subject*, pp. 247–258. Edited by Paul, C. and Thomson-Salo, F. London: Karnac Books.

Perelberg, R.J. (2015). *Murdered Father, Dead Father*. London and New York: Routledge.

Pozzi, M. (2003). *Psychic Hooks and Bolts*. London: Karnac Books.

Raphael-Leff, J. (2003). *Parent-Infant Psychodynamics*. London and Philadelphia: Whurr Publications.

Shakespeare, W. (1596–9). The Merchant of Venice. 2ii. In: *The Complete Work of William Shakespeare.*, p. 222. Edited by Dover Wilson, J. London: Octopus Books Limited.

Trowell, J., and Etchegoyen, A. (2002). *The Importance of Fathers*. Hove: Brunner-Routledge.

Vallino, D. (2004). *Essere Neonati*. Roma: Borla.

Von Klitzing, K., Simoni, H., Amsler, F., and Burgin, D. (1999). The Role of the Father in Early Family Interaction. *Infant Mental Health Journal*, Vol. 20: 222–237.

10 Breaking the cycle

Dreamy and distracted,
You stumbled upon the Friend.
You felt His presence
And froze on your path.
If you don't have
The strength to face Him,
Why seek the circle of the Drunks?
                    Rumi, circa 1250, p. 57

The literature

Klein (1927) writes that even the quite small child, after showing his most sadistic impulses in his play and drawing, acts his "greatest capacity for love and the wish to make all possible sacrifices to be loved" (p. 176). In 1929, she writes about the creative work ensuing from the suicidal depression of painter Ruth Kjär; "the desire to make reparation, to make good the injury psychologically done to the mother and also to restore herself was at the bottom of the compelling urge to paint" (p. 218). Regarding children, she writes:

> When in the course of its analysis, the child begins to show stronger constructive tendencies in all sorts of ways in its play and its sublimations [...] it also exhibits changes in its relation to its father or mother, or to its brothers and sisters [...], improved object relationship in general, and a growth of social feeling.
>
> (Klein, 1933, p. 255)

Hinshelwood (1991) writes:

> Reparation comes out of the real concern for the object, a pining for it. It may involve great self-sacrifice in the external world into which damaged objects have been projected. Powerful reparative urges are often responsible for lives devoted to humanitarian ends and lived in great hardship.
>
> (p. 415)

He continues:

> Reparation, though it is concerned primarily with the state of the internal world and good object that forms the core of the personality, is usually expressed in actions towards objects in the external world which represents the damaged internal object, or which can be introjected in phantasy to support the internal world. It is thus a force for constructive action in the external world.
>
> (pp. 415–6)

John Byng-Hall (1995) writes:

> Family scripts can be defined as the family's shared expectations of how family roles are to be performed within various contexts. […] Family members can identify themselves with particular roles, as well as become identified by others as characteristically occupying those roles. […] For example, children can vow to themselves to follow different patterns when they become parents. No one, however, acts in a way that successfully breaks the current pattern. Hence, family expectations of what will happen remain the same.
>
> (p. 4)

"The therapist can help to create a new coconstructed scenario by suggesting a goal […] which the family then achieves in their own way […] rewriting their own [script]" (p. 7). "Choosing a partner with whom to start a family usually involves the opportunity to reenact both replicative and corrective scripts, in ways that repeat the best of both parents' experience" (p. 43).

Several parents I have written about in this book also wanted to give their infants different experiences from those they had had and this is not an uncommon reason for seeking help. Amongst several parents, I have chosen Siobhan, who was very conscious about not repeating her past and being determined to re-write her own story and break through her family cycle. This was her major, conscious aim, within an almost ideal relationship with her baby.

Clinical vignette

Siobhan, Paolo and baby Felix

Siobhan was determined to break the cycle of intergenerational family abuses of all sorts: physical, sexual and substance abuse being perpetuated on all the children in her family for at least the last two generations, so she said. She was pregnant for the first time with a good man, different from the previous, violent one: she had begun separating from her family with some success. Never having benefited from counselling before, she asked to try it to help her move away from an unsound family history. She knew she could not do it alone. She was referred to a parent-infant psychotherapy service. There we met.

Her baby was two months old, sturdy, dark haired and smiling when we first met at the Centre.

She was very open with me from the start and recounted a childhood and adolescence history of neglect and abuse by damaged alcoholic parents and a violent boyfriend. The neglect and abuse were repeated even by the hand of the foster carers, who were meant to look after her when she left her parental home. Eventually she and her older sister – a helpful figure of her early years – were adopted but as soon as they were old enough, they moved out separately to be on their own.

This story was told with a great deal of self-consciousness, anger at the failing parents, at the now-dead father in particular, sadness at having had a rough deal, but also guilt for having been the one who was better off in her family. Her sister was spoken of warmly and gratefully and it was her care that most likely propelled Siobhan to want to break off from past, abusive experiences.

In the session she needed to show me the best of herself as a mother: she placed baby Felix on a cushion on the mat with a bottle in his hands for him to feed himself. She said she wanted him to become independent soon. She kept anxiously wiping the ordinary dribbling milk off his mouth even when it was not needed. I became concerned about possible maternal projections on him: was his ordinary need for milk seen as greed that needed bridling? Was his dribbling mouth, that she constantly wiped, a reminder of her alcoholic, dribbling parents? I had to help her see Felix as a baby in his own right and not be confused with alcoholic adults. She was able to accept both my idea that babies need holding by a caring mother-figure when feeding, and the link between ordinary baby dribbling and alcoholics' dribbling.

She had more memories about witnessing domestic violence and feelings of guilt for being spared abuse – to some extent – in comparison to her many siblings and half siblings. Feeling she had been more fortunate than them propelled her to want to be a better mother and to help her own mother and siblings; but this was really not understood by her entrenched family and was very disappointing to Siobhan.

When I felt that she was skidding on painful memories and stopped being there with Felix, I introduced mindfulness and encouraged her to breathe consciously while focusing on her body sensations and on her baby. A moment of pause and bodily awareness of herself and of her baby was needed. She would practice it at home when anxious or stressed – she said.

Felix was a handsome, well looked-after and loved baby: in the session he lay alert on his back on the mat, looking at, and following our faces and motions, as if taking part in the conversation and in the environment. When painful memories and accounts were told, he regurgitated his milk and cried, while his Mum was too absorbed in her unheard childhood suffering and tears to be able to tune in with him. Talking to him in a soothing tone of voice and describing what he might be feeling, calmed him down at last. The deep and calm sound of my words had a similar effect to that of a mantra on a meditating adult.

We danced through moments of frustration when my comments were hardly kept in mind and I was to feel the irritation and annoyance that Siobhan had felt and was still undoubtedly feeling towards adult figures in her life.

Siobhan eventually modified both her occasionally impatient response to Felix and became less cut-off, more able to observe him and to hold him physically.

Just as Felix's feeding was suddenly stopped to burp him or wipe his mouth, so were our sessions, which were often cancelled due to illnesses or to family commitments such as the death of beloved relatives. We had to be aware of "addiction" not only to alcohol but also to our session: weekly sessions were too frequent and to seductive to Siobhan. But she always came back determined to give Felix a better life and to continue our work together. His father, whom I never met – and his loving extended family abroad – were an important source of strength for her and for him.

I was to leave the service after about nine months of work with them. The promise to stay in touch with me afterwards was not kept nor did a proper, formal goodbye session happen. This was due to the death of somebody else in her family and to a deep-rooted difficulty in facing ending, separation and death which were acted out by Siobhan in sessions, leaving me alone to process them.

I had the good fortune to meet Siobhan and Felix again, when he was two-and-a-half and for the purpose of showing her what I had written on our earlier psychotherapy. The visit took place in their home and Felix, a handsome, dark-haired child, was very excited and chatted non-stop with mum and me. He showed me his toys, when asked to do so, played for a short while then chucked them around mischievously. Siobhan took him in her stride, talked with him warmly and disciplined him when necessary: he responded well but also tried her boundaries.

Siobhan was working part-time feeling settled but hoping to move house in the near future and, in the far future, to move with Felix's father to his country of origin. This sounded a good, hopeful plan for the whole family. Her relationship with her own family was boundaried and self-protective and she felt that Felix was the most important thing in her life. She was proud for having broken the cycle of the unhealthy lifestyle of her original family.

Bibliography

Byng-Hall, J. (1995). *Rewriting Family Scripts*. New York: The Guilford Press.

Hinshelwood, R.D. (1991). *A Dictionary of Kleinian Thought*. London: Free Association Books.

Klein, M. (1927). Criminal Tendencies in Normal Children. In: *Love, Guilt And Reparation*, pp. 170–185, Edited by: M. Masud and R. Khan. London: The Hogarth Press, 1975.

Klein, M. (1929). Infantile Anxiety-Situations Reflected in a Work of Art and in the Creative Impulse. In: *Love, Guilt and Reparation*, pp. 210–218. London: The Hogarth Press, 1975.

Klein, M. (1933). The Early Development of Conscience in the Child. In: *Love, Guilt and Reparation*, pp. 248–257, Edited by: M. Masud and R. Khan. London: The Hogarth Press, 1975.

Rumi. (circa 1250). *Rumi's Little Book of the HEART*, p. 57. Edited by: Mafi, M. and Melita Kolin, A. Charlottesville, VA: Hampton Roads Publishing Company, Inc.

Wax, R. (2018). Kids. In: *How to Be Human*, pp. 115–142, Edited by: R. Wax. UK: Penguin Random House.

Index